Autism: A Very Short Introduction

Titles in the series include the following:

Uta Frith

AUTISM

A Very Short Introduction

OXFORD
UNIVERSITY PRESS

OXFORD
UNIVERSITY PRESS

Great Clarendon Street, Oxford OX2 6DP

Oxford University Press is a department of the University of Oxford.
It furthers the University's objective of excellence in research, scholarship,
and education by publishing worldwide in

Oxford New York

Auckland Cape Town Dar es Salaam Hong Kong Karachi
Kuala Lumpur Madrid Melbourne Mexico City Nairobi
New Delhi Shanghai Taipei Toronto

With offices in

Argentina Austria Brazil Chile Czech Republic France Greece
Guatemala Hungary Italy Japan Poland Portugal Singapore
South Korea Switzerland Thailand Turkey Ukraine Vietnam

Oxford is a registered trade mark of Oxford University Press
in the UK and in certain other countries

Published in the United States
by Oxford University Press Inc., New York

British Library Cataloguing in Publication Data

Data available

Library of Congress Cataloging in Publication Data

Frith, Uta.
Autism : a very short introduction / Uta Frith.
    p.   cm. – (Very short introductions (VSI))
            ISBN 978-0-19-920756-5
        1. Autism in children.   I. Title.
            RJ506.A9.F694   2008
618.92′89–dc22   2008027742

ISBN 978-0-19-920756-5

Typeset by SPI Publisher Services, Pondicherry, India
Printed and bound by
CPI Group (UK) Ltd, Croydon, CR0 4YY

Contents

Acknowledgements

I thought this short introduction would be quick and easy to write. How wrong! It was a long, slow and sometimes uncomfortable process. It made me revisit my past and review different ideas about autism, having to make selections as well as omissions. It made me realize that there are rather few solid facts about autism. Instead, I have selected what I consider good bets about the results of still ongoing research. I am hopeful that the studies I have picked will stand the test of time.

Given these difficulties it was imperative that I had knowledgeable reviewers. I was very fortunate to count Chris Frith, Francesca Happé, and Sarah White among them. They gave invaluable advice and critically important suggestions for improvement. They did not discourage me from including some more speculative thoughts.

I would also like to thank my most constant and constructive critics, Alex and Martin Frith. Alex edited most of the chapters in a sensitive and accomplished manner. My friend, Heide Grieve, as always gave excellent advice. I am deeply grateful to Chris, Franky and Sarah for helping me to decide what should be included in this introduction to autism and what could be left out. This book belongs to them.

Aarhus, 24 January 2008

List of illustrations

9 Sally–Anne test **68**
This test was used by
Baron-Cohen, S., Leslie, A.
and Frith, U. (1985) *Cognition*,
21, 37–46

10 Triangles interacting **70**
Adapted from Castelli, F., Happé, F.,
Frith, U. and Frith, C.D. (2000)
Neuroimage 12, 3, 314–25

11 The brain's mentalizing
system **71**
Adapted from Castelli, F., Happé, F.,
Frith, U. and Frith, C.D. (2000)
Neuroimage 12, 3, 314–25

12 Patterns of eye gaze **75**
From Klin, A., Jones, W., Schultz, R.,
Volkmar, F., and Cohen, D. (2002)
American Journal of Psychiatry, 159,
895–908. Reprinted with permission
from American Psychiatric
Association

13 Imitation of hand
movements **78**
Based on Hamilton, A.F.d.C.,
Brindley, R.M., Frith, U. (2007)
Neuropsychologia, 45, 1859–68.
Photo courtesy of Antonia Hamilton

14 Contagious yawning **80**
Copyright Digital Vision/Alamy;
From Senju A., Maeda M., Kikuchi Y.,
Hasegawa T., Tojo and Osanai H.
(2007) *Biological Letters*, 22, 706–8.
Reprinted with permission from the
Royal Society

15 London cityscape, by Stephen
Wiltshire **86**
© Stephen Wiltshire

16 Attention to detail **89**
© John Birdsall

17 Tasks showing superior
performance **92**
From Dakin, S. & Frith, U. (2005)
Vagaries of visual perception in
autism. *Neuron*, 48, 497–507.
Reprinted with permission from Cell
Press

18 In the supermarket **97**
© Left Lane Productions/Corbis

19 Temple Grandin **113**
© Rosalie Winard

20 Thomas the Tank Engine **116**
© Gullane (Thomas) LLC 2003.
Published by Egmunt UK Ltd. and
used with permission

The publisher and the author apologize for any errors or omissions in the above list. If contacted they will be pleased to rectify these at the earliest opportunity.

Chapter 1
The autism spectrum

Is it autism?

Imagine a young mother and her baby. She adores him, and he is gorgeous. But, deep down Diane can't help worrying just occasionally, whether Mickey will grow up a normal happy boy. How could she tell if he has autism, for example? There is so much about autism in the news. Almost one in a hundred children born are autistic with five times as many boys as girls. An autistic child conjures up all sorts of scenarios, most of them bleak. And what are the first signs of autism? Is it significant that Mickey cries a lot, doesn't sleep much and is not easily calmed? Lots of babies are like that, Diane's mother says. She worries, however, that Mickey does not always turn around when she calls him from across the room.

When Diane started to read about autism she found the information quite unsettling. She read that some children are very delayed in their general development. Then there were some children who gave no cause for concern at all until well into their second year of life. One child never spoke; another was actually a little genius. Diane, like many people who are starting to find out about autism, is perplexed, but also intrigued.

The enigma of autism

When I first started to study autism as a young student in London in the 1960s I too was perplexed and intrigued. More than that, I was utterly fascinated as well as puzzled by the children I saw at London's Maudsley Hospital, where I trained to be a clinical psychologist. Because of this fascination I never worked as a clinical psychologist, but became a research scientist instead. But of course, fascination is not enough. At that time the Maudsley hospital housed four of the pioneers of autism research: child psychiatrist Michael Rutter, epidemiologist Lorna Wing, and psychologists Neil O'Connor and Beate Hermelin. I had read some of their papers, but did not even realize that they worked at the same place.

The papers reported ingenious experiments on perception and memory. They compared children who were then labelled mentally retarded and children then just beginning to be labelled autistic, and they found clear differences between the groups. These differences were clues to different minds. They could not be trivially explained by lack of intelligence or lack of motivation. I was completely bowled over by the fact that such elegant experiments could be done and gave such clear results. Beate Hermelin and Neil O'Connor had already worked out ways of answering questions that puzzled me deeply. For example, why do some tasks, apparently simple, seem quite impossible for autistic children? Why are they doing well on other tasks, which appear difficult for others? Why is a child who has a good memory for words unable to comprehend their meaning? I now believe that it was just these paradoxes and puzzles that cast something of a spell on me. They kept urging me to find solutions.

Forty years later, the spell is still powerful. Although there are answers to some of these questions—and we will explore them in this book—there is much more still to be discovered, and the puzzle of autism is far from being solved.

What I learned right at the beginning is that with autism nothing is what it seems at first glance. Just because a child with autism doesn't respond to your overtures, doesn't mean that the child rejects you. The reasons for not responding are much deeper. Further, just because a child can remember words and pictures does not mean that they can remember names and faces of people. One of the most startling realizations that hit me was that being autistic could be in many ways worse than being born blind or deaf. Autistic children—barring exceptions—can see and hear, often exquisitely well. But, while blind and deaf children can still receive and respond to social signals through a special sense, autistic children don't have this sense.

It is hard to imagine what it is like *not* to have a social sense, *not* to be tuned in to other people, their actions, reactions, and the signals they give out to you and each other. As it is, autistic children are not tuned into these things. However, they do have mental capacities that help them to learn about these signals. But they learn in a different way. Sadly, the knowledge they acquire is not the same as the ordinary 'tuned in' knowledge that we all take for granted. A colour-blind person can acquire knowledge of colours and name them correctly, but their experience of colours will remain different. So it is with autism and the experience of social communication.

Why does learning in autism proceed along a different route? Because autism starts so early in life, many of the social routes to learning about the world are blocked. Normally developing children can easily follow the path that has been carved out by evolution and culture. But autistic children have to find their own special routes on the byways. This makes them very different from each other as well as different from children who do not have autism.

The autism spectrum

When I first saw autistic children I was only dimly aware that autism comes in degrees, from mild to severe. Actually, all the cases I saw were severe. When I see autistic children now, I am still surprised at how many cases are high functioning and how many cases have only mild and moderate degrees of autism. To see a child with classic autism has become the exception. But I am reassured that such cases are still there, and that they have the same features as they did forty years ago. However, autism is no longer a narrow category but has widened enormously to embrace a whole range of autistic conditions. It has now become generally accepted to talk about an autism spectrum.

What is meant by this spectrum? Actually, it hides a vast array of 'autisms'. All the autisms originate from before birth, and all affect the developing brain. However, their effect on the developing mind can be very different. Consequently, there is a vastly different range of behaviours. Sometimes a family can be justly proud of their child, who is interestingly different, and possibly gifted in some special way. Sometimes a family will be destroyed because their child will be so difficult to manage that they simply cannot cope. Of course there are many shades in between, and most cases come with a mixture of rewarding and fascinating as well as aggravating and challenging features.

Every individual is unique in a multitude of ways, but they also resemble each other in some fundamental preferences and characteristics. What binds them all together, the mild and severe forms of the spectrum? At the core, there is always a characteristic inability to engage in ordinary reciprocal social interaction. There is also a characteristic rigidity of behaviour, with a multitude of consequences. That is why no one has yet given up the idea that there is a common pattern behind the kaleidoscope of individual behaviours. I will therefore frequently use the familiar terms autism and autistic, as a reminder that there is central idea behind the spectrum.

Three cases

Now we shall look at three cases closely based on real cases from different parts of the autism spectrum. David has classic autism. Gary has an autism spectrum disorder (ASD) with a diffuse and atypical picture, but such complex cases are actually quite common. Edward has classic Asperger syndrome.

David

David was 3 when he was diagnosed as autistic. At that time he hardly looked at people, was not talking, and seemed lost in his own world. He loved to bounce on a trampoline for hours and was extremely adept at doing jigsaw puzzles. At 10 years of age David had developed well physically, but emotionally remained very immature. He had a beautiful face with delicate features. Family life has always had to fit around David, not the other way round. He was and still is extremely stubborn in his likes and dislikes. At one stage he only ate yoghurt and refused all other kinds of food. More often than not his mother has to give in to his urgent and repeated demands, which easily escalate into tantrums.

David learned to talk when he was 5. He now goes to a special school for autistic children, where he is happy. He has a daily routine, which he never varies. It is hard to tell how intelligent David is. Some things he learns with great skill and speed. For example, he learned to read all by himself. He now reads fluently, but he doesn't understand what he reads. He also loves to do sums. However, he has been extremely slow to learn other skills, for example, eating at the family table, or getting dressed. David has an excellent memory. He imitates what he hears very precisely and has a beautiful singing voice. He also has perfect pitch.

David is now 12 years old. He still does not spontaneously play with other children. He has obvious difficulties in communicating with other people who don't know him well. With those who do know him, he communicates entirely on his own terms. He makes no concessions to their wishes or interests and cannot take onboard another person's point of view. In this way David is indifferent to the social world and continues to live in a world of his own.

Gary

When Gary was at primary school an experienced teacher observed that he had unusual problems in communicating with other children and could not manage to work in a group in class. Gary's parents accepted these problems as part of his personality. He seemed to be a very obstinate child, and happy to play computer games for hours. Referred to an educational psychologist by the school when problems with Gary seemed only to get worse, he was eventually seen at a clinic at age 12. The psychologist explained that Gary had a Pervasive Developmental Disorder, a category that includes autism, Asperger syndrome, and a few other rare conditions. Actually Gary was diagnosed as having PDD-NOS, Pervasive Developmental Disorder—Not Otherwise Specified. This is a category for cases that have autistic features, but not all features are necessarily present. The psychologist also mentioned Asperger syndrome when she talked to Gary's parents. They immediately favoured this label as it helped them to explain Gary's problems to other people.

The psychological assessments showed that Gary also had attention deficit disorder, and dyspraxia, as evident in his clumsiness on motor tasks. His main problems, however, were poor communication skills and an inability to understand other people. Gary was placed in a succession of different schools. In each case he was said to be difficult and disruptive. He bitterly complained about being bullied. Sadly, he was. However, Gary's classmates made some efforts to understand him. But they failed because Gary could not tell the difference between being teased or criticized.

Gary is now in his twenties and lives at home. So far, he has shown little interest in his mother's suggestions for finding a job and still spends most of his time playing computer games. Gary often says that he would like to have a girlfriend. On one occasion he had started to follow an attractive young woman everywhere, waiting outside her house for hours, but never talking to her. Now Gary's family are watching carefully for signs of inappropriate social behaviour. At his mother's insistence, Gary has joined a social skills group for people with Asperger syndrome, and he now attends the monthly meetings without fail.

Edward

Edward was diagnosed as having Asperger syndrome at the age of 8. Although clearly very bright, his teacher felt at her wits end with him. She said that she could not teach him, and that instead he taught himself, but only what he wanted to learn. He could not make any attempts to fit in with ordinary classroom activities and he refused point blank to follow the set curriculum. Edward's family had not realized the extent of this problem. On the contrary, they had always thought of Edward as an extraordinarily gifted child. By 5 years of age he had acquired an astounding vocabulary, mainly by reading dictionaries. He was rather fearful of playing with other children, but relished the attention he got from adults. His family dotes on him and he seems to share a lot of interests and mannerisms with his father. Both are bookish people and can talk very persistently about their interests. Edward started to collect birds' eggs from about the age of 4 and has developed an intricate system for classifying them.

Edward is now 20 years old and is about to study maths at a top university. He went to a private school where the teachers were sympathetic and let him follow his own interests. At school he obtained excellent marks in all science subjects. Other subjects simply did not interest him. He proclaimed loudly that literature was a waste of time. Apart from being in the chess club, he never became part of a circle of friends. Outwardly, Edward dismisses all social events as a bore. He is fluent when he talks with his father and corresponds with ornithologists all over the world, but seems to be tongue tied when faced with people his own age. Edward sticks out in a crowd, not only by his tall and lanky appearance, but also by his mannerisms and loud high-pitched voice. However, he has started to read books of manners and body language and is hoping they will improve his social skills.

Edward is very knowledgeable about Asperger syndrome and avidly participates in Asperger discussion forums on the web. He knows that he is far more intelligent than most 'neurotypicals'. However, there are signs that Edward is often anxious and sometimes depressed, and he is being seen by a psychiatrist who will carefully monitor him in the transition period when he leaves home to go to college.

The three core features of the autism spectrum

The examples of David, Gary, and Edward show how enormously varied the core signs of autism are, at least on the surface. Therefore, a lot of clinical experience is needed to make a diagnosis. The behaviour of each individual differs according to so many factors that they are difficult to list, but they include at least age, family background, general ability, education, and the child's own temperament and personality. Nevertheless, there is common ground. These are the core features of the autism spectrum, the chief diagnostic criteria. You can find them on several helpful websites. Here we unpack their meaning using our example cases.

The first of the core features of ASD concerns **reciprocal social interaction**. It is not enough to be a loner, to behave embarrassingly, or to be clumsy in social situations. The difficulty reveals itself most acutely in peer interactions. At young ages, this means other children—not adults. Adults often make huge allowances to smooth over awkward social situations. A clear sign of failing reciprocal interaction is a lack of engagement with other children.

In the case of David, the failure in social interaction can at first glance be described as a lack of social interest, or aloofness as regards other people. However, this aloofness is actually an inability to engage with others, even to the extent that he never asked to be taught to read, but taught himself. Gary is unable to read the social signals of others. He has no idea how to get a girlfriend although he would very much like to have one. Edward can socially interact with people who appreciate his intelligence, but avoids social interaction with his peers. He tries to find out about social rules.

The second related core feature concerns **communication**. Deep down, the ability to communicate hinges on a message being acknowledged as happening. One person needs to wish to communicate, and the other needs to wish to receive the communication. Communication does not have to be spoken words, but can be gestures or facial expressions. Without the signs that accompany sending and receiving a message, there can be no true communication.

David has the most severe problems in communication. He spoke late and his use of language is extremely limited, that is, he uses it if he wants something, but not to express feelings or thoughts. Gary has more subtle difficulties. He finds it impossible to know whether people make jokes from the way they talk, and feels rebuffed when he tries to talk to others. Edward is highly articulate, but he does not enjoy ordinary chitchat. His ability to engage in a two-way conversation has improved since he has started systematically to gather information about

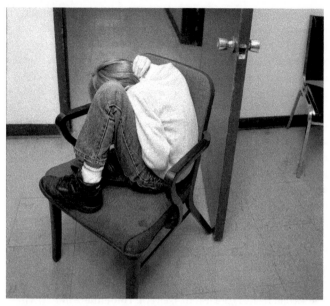

1a. Key feature 1: In a world of his own

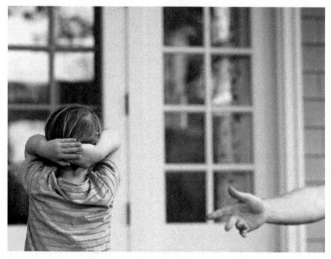

1b. Key feature 2: Unable to communicate

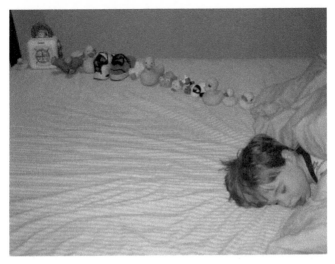

1c. Key feature 3: Restricted and repetitive. Lining up toys as seen in this charming picture has often been observed in young autistic children's play

communication, through reading books on etiquette and body language and through reading about Asperger syndrome.

The third core feature is of a different kind from the first two: it is about **repetitive activities and narrow interests**. What is *autistic* about these features, which seem not unfamiliar to many parents of young children? Lining blocks or cars up in neat little patterns may be cute just once or twice, but it becomes very sad when this is done day after day without exploring other possibilities of playing with blocks or cars. It is the extreme nature of the repetitions and the obsessive quality of the interests that are typical of autism. Another way to look at repetitive behaviour is to think of it as extreme stubbornness. In fact there is a strong resistance to change and an aversion to novelty. Doing the same thing, exactly the same thing, watching the same video, eating the same food, day after day, is the kind of excessive pattern that is

11

found in autistic children. It is often less noticeable in autistic adults, where the behavioural repertoire has widened through learning and experience.

David's love of bouncing is an example of repetitive action and his interest in print and reading was described as obsessive. Gary did not have this feature and this made his diagnosis less straightforward. His interest in computer games was not really different from that of other young people. Edward had a number of different intensely pursued interests in succession. At one point he abandoned his interest in dictionaries and took up maths instead.

The pictures on the preceding pages show examples of what it is that clinicians focus on as significant signs or symptoms of autism in the childhood years. In the next chapter we will look at how some of the behavioural signs change with age.

Everyone agrees that autism is a developmental disorder. Development means change, and in autism it usually means improvement, an increasing ability to cope with the frightening aspects of a world that is not shared and therefore unpredictable. The repetitive and obsessive features often also fade to have a less severe impact on life. These improvements can all be expected when there is good education and support for the growing child and his or her family.

When does autism start?

This is a long and complicated story, as yet unreadable to us. Autism has its origin well before birth. At some point, a tiny fault occurs. This fault is somewhere in the genetic programme that results in a human being, with its enormously complex central nervous system. This fault is so subtle that for the most part the programme runs off smoothly, and a baby is born who looks perfectly healthy. Only from about the second year of life do the consequences of the tiny fault emerge with rather major and sometimes devastating effects.

Why only then? Perhaps, this point in time is critical for the foundation of typically human social behaviour, more critical even than the social interest that is already there in the first year. This is worth dwelling on. The healthy newborn infant, straight from birth, shows strong signs of social interest. For instance, babies prefer to look at a face rather than at a pattern, and a real face rather than a scrambled face; they prefer direct eye contact to averted eyes. They prefer to listen to speech rather than scrambled sounds; they turn to people, smile at people, show responses to familiar adults that are different from strangers, and so on.

Babies are such powerfully social creatures for a reason. For thousands of years of evolution babies have utterly depended on other human beings for their survival. And yet, the social gifts they manifest so early are quite one-sided. They cry, they look, they smile, and they babble. All these behaviours act as powerful social signals for the mother. Crying, for example, will ensure that the baby gets food and comfort. However, it seems that there is a step change in human social development at the end of the first year of life. It goes together with a step change in general physical and mental development. The baby starts to walk and to talk. Something happens that lifts the already flourishing but perhaps mainly one-sided interaction onto a different level where interactions are truly reciprocal. And here lies the core social problem in autism.

Everyone can see that in the first year of life a baby grows in size and weight at amazing speed, but we can't see how its brain grows. Almost all the nerve cells of the brain are already there at birth; it is the connections between the nerve cells that grow so phenomenally. The system is being wired up with millions and millions of connectors (synapses) and connecting fibres. The brain's communication highways are being constructed. This construction also includes eliminating bad or unnecessary connections. As the baby turns into a toddler, there is a major reorganization of the brain, and with it is a major change in the way the child interacts with other human beings.

Given that autism has social impairments at its core, one might expect that these impairments should be obvious even in the first year of life. It is remarkable that they are not. It is generally in the second year that autistic development starts to deviate from the norm, not in the first. Autistic babies seemingly stay behind and do not make the vital step change in social interaction towards true joint interaction.

What is joint attention?

There is attention from one individual to another and there is joint attention where two individuals are deliberately and simultaneously attending to an object. This accomplishment is thought by many to be the basis of true reciprocal interaction and, however social the baby is from birth, joint attention is not shown until the end of the first year of life or even later. Lack of joint attention in a toddler is a worrying sign of autism. At the same time, it is a behaviour that is difficult to induce in children who do not show it spontaneously. What constitutes joint attention?

One individual can draw the attention of another to share interest in an object and this shared interest is in itself enjoyable. Eye gaze can direct attention, and so can pointing with a finger and showing an object. One of the earliest signs of autism is that the child shows little sign of trying to attract the attention of another person by look or gesture. Instead the child appears to be oblivious to the other person present. In fact, autistic children are not oblivious. They are of course utterly dependent on other people and rely on them to have their desires and needs fulfilled. Indeed, the child can show this dependence in a most pathetic way, for instance by crying disconsolately or by dragging a person by the hand to a place where they hope to get what they need. These apparently desperate attempts seem strange to parents, when they would be only too ready to help the child if only the child gave them a small hint. But this is exactly what the autistic child can't do. He or she cannot elicit the attention in what seems to everyone a perfectly simple and obvious way, for instance by seeking eye contact and trying to engage the adult by simple gestures.

And yet it is difficult to recognize the absence of these signs. Sometimes children who have perfectly healthy brains are slow at developing social skills. Children's temperament and social interests differ, and some are slow at learning to speak. This was the case with Mickey. As a baby he did not show a lot of social interest and sometimes he seemed oblivious when called by name. This was worrying. However, on his second birthday he gave clear signs of joint attention. When his grandmother visited, he held up his new teddy to her and laughed when she pretended to talk to the teddy.

Regression or lack of progress?

Alice reported that her son Tom had spoken very early. His first words, at the age of 10 months were 'car, plane, bike'. He was a healthy and happy baby, walking at 10 months and exploring his environment with great energy like any other toddler. He acquired at least another dozen words, but from about eighteen months Tom seemed to become more absorbed with himself, and it gradually dawned on Alice that he never spoke any more. He seemed to have lost interest in his surroundings and did not progress like other toddlers. A year later Tom was diagnosed autistic with regressive development. Alice learned that this pattern of sad decline was quite frequent, and there was nothing and nobody that could be blamed for the autism. At least 30 per cent of parents have this experience.

The question is whether there is actually a decline and a regression? Or, is it more a lack of progress towards another stage of development? Could it be that Tom was like other children at first, but then other children zoomed ahead, because they had entered a new phase of mental development? Alice thought she noticed a distinct change, and she agonized about what might have triggered this change in Tom. She could simply not accept that a perfectly normal baby, who showed plentiful signs of social interest, should suddenly start behaving like an autistic child. Something must have happened: perhaps an unnoticed brain disease, perhaps some kind of poisoning from a substance that may be harmless to others. This is almost certainly not the case for Tom. Actually, it is extremely rare that autism is caused by some external agent. However, only solid research about the actual course of development of the brain in autism will remove these inevitable worries.

The case of Patricia was quite different. She was always concerned that there was something wrong. Her daughter Sylvia was a restless and difficult baby who cried a lot and slept very little. She played intensely with her rattle and gazed at the pattern of the curtains with her big beautiful eyes. During the second year, it became abundantly clear to Patricia that other children of Sylvia's age were a long way ahead in their development. While Sylvia was physically progressing very well, mentally she seemed to stay very much as she had been as a baby. Her interests in particular toys became even more intense and it was difficult to attract her attention away from them. She never seemed to look at people. She only turned to others when she needed something that instant. She never looked at her dolls and teddies either. She turned away when other children came and invited her to play. Other children pointed to objects and pictures in books and rapidly learned their names. Sylvia did none of these things.

Patricia reported later that she had hoped that Sylvia's difficulties as a baby were somehow to do with colic or teething and would go away once she was older. The frequent crying did go away, but Sylvia continued to be a poor sleeper. Patricia was rightly alarmed when Sylvia did not show interest in other children and did not pick up language.

Alice and Patricia had very different experiences with their children. But it turned out later that the development of both Tom and Sylvia was not actually very dissimilar. Both were given help from a speech therapist and both eventually learned to talk. Their mental development improved by leaps and bounds when they attended a specialist school.

What about little Mickey? Not all children are equally sociable and they don't develop equally fast. Mickey did learn to speak quite late, but he turned out to be a very friendly but occasionally shy little boy with a lot of imagination and a dry sense of humour. Diane was able to put her worries about autism aside, when Mickey entered nursery school. She could see that he fitted in with the other children, playing in the playhouse, and taking his beloved teddy for a picnic together with his friends' teddies. When she came to fetch him he rushed to show her the pictures he had made that day.

Why did Diane have to worry for so long? And why did Patricia have to wait for a couple of years before Sylvia was diagnosed?

How early can we push the diagnosis of autism?

As long as the diagnosis of autism is based on behaviour, a definitive pronouncement can only be made with hindsight. Perhaps, once a biological test is available, the diagnosis can be made before birth, but such a test still seems far in the future. Having to rely on behavioural criteria means having to live with ambiguity. And because the range of differences *between* all children is so large, even experienced clinicians can make misjudgements when pressed for a categorical pronouncement too early.

What happens when parents seek professional help, when the social and emotional development of their child seems to deteriorate or simply not move on? In the past there has often been a long and sometimes harrowing road, but now health professionals are more knowledgeable about autistic disorders and highly aware of the need for early intervention. Ideally, an experienced clinician will interview the parents about their child's development in detail, and will also test and observe the child. Then provision can be made for a programme of special education to start right away. For this reason it is important that this diagnosis is done as early as possible.

However, there is a dilemma. Researchers asked the question: if a child is diagnosed at the age of 24 months, how certain is the diagnosis? Researchers investigated how likely it is that the diagnosis is confirmed two years later. They showed that in the majority of cases the diagnosis was indeed confirmed, but still one-third of the cases were eventually not considered autistic. The study also showed that there is almost complete certainty about the diagnosis when the child is older than 30 months.

Many people feel that despite the risk of false alarms, early diagnosis is a desirable aim. One interesting solution to the problem is to proceed in two stages. At the first stage, around the age of 18 months, there could be screening for all children. At the second stage, perhaps around 30 months, a full diagnostic assessment could be offered to those children who had raised concerns. In fact, a screening instrument has already been developed. Three signs are assessed. First, does the child show 'joint attention', such as pointing with a finger. Second, is he or she following an adult's gaze. Third, does he or she engage in simple pretend play? Most typically developing children aged 18 months can master these things. Most autistic children can't. However, a number of children who apparently show these key behaviours nevertheless later go on to have an autistic disorder. This is likely to be Asperger syndrome.

In the next chapter we will consider some of the historical reasons for how we think of autism now. We will also look at the changes in what autism looks like over the course of a child's development into adulthood.

Chapter 2
The changing face of autism

A little bit of history

A hundred years ago, autism was not heard of. The name didn't
exist. Of course, the condition existed, and there is some evidence
for this from centuries past. However, documents that give
detailed descriptions of likely cases are very scarce. The two people
who named the condition were Leo Kanner (1894–1981) and Hans
Asperger (1906–80), and they did it simultaneously in the early
1940s right in the middle of the Second World War. At that time
the attention of most people was elsewhere; indeed the world was
in chaos. The general recovery from the war took until the late
1950s and 1960s, and at this time, a handful of parents and a
handful of professionals began to recognize autism in children.
This started first in Europe and the USA and spread sporadically
to other parts of the world. However, it took another thirty years
for the general public to have heard of autism through the media.

The history of autism remains to be told. Kanner's inspiring
portrayal of the features of autism had extraordinary impact.
These children were beautiful, they had talents, but they also were
severely disturbed and had serious learning problems. With these
puzzling features it is not surprising that a powerful myth arose.
This is how it goes: some children experience a rejection so
traumatic that there is no way but to withdraw from the hostile

world outside. This withdrawal is so complete that nothing can reverse it, except lengthy psychotherapy. Only, psychotherapy did not produce the desired effects. Gradually some practical ideas spread and succeeded in improving the quality of life of the children as well as their families. The most beneficial and perhaps also most obvious of these ideas was special education.

In 1964, Bernard Rimland's book on autism was a breath of fresh air. It championed an approach that had already been adopted by scientists at a number of medical and psychological centres. These scientists analysed cognitive abilities of autistic children, such as speech and language, perception and memory, in detail. They found strengths as well as weaknesses, and this overturned two ideas: one, that autistic children were mentally retarded overall; the other, that they were secretly highly intelligent. Clearly, they were a bit of both, and this paradoxical pattern seems to be a hallmark of autism. In 1971 the *Journal for Autism and Childhood Schizophrenia* was first published, now known as the *Journal for Autism and Developmental Disorders*. At that time autism was still little known and believed to be very rare. Nobody guessed then that in the future there would be so much interest and so many research reports that several other specialist journals would be founded.

Not only did research efforts increase, the numbers of cases increased massively too. All this went hand in hand with the increase in the awareness of autism and the widening of the boundaries of the autism spectrum. From the 1990s Asperger syndrome became a familiar label. The prototype of Asperger syndrome is the highly intelligent individual who has social impairments as well as abstruse interests. This new prototype was soon mixed up with older stereotypes of the mad genius. An idea that took off at amazing speed was that many of us, and men in particular, have autistic features. Namely, they lack social sensitivity and have obsessive interests. The boundaries of the autistic spectrum are still in flux. Will there be a clear line to distinguish autistic disorders from variants of perfectly normal differences in personality? This is one of the questions that now need to be resolved.

At the feet of the great pioneers

To me it feels that I have experienced a large part of this history personally during my own life. I have taken on board the changes in the concept of autism and have observed the huge increase in numbers of children and adults diagnosed autistic. From being unknown and obscure, autism has become a familiar topic.

I received my first introduction to autism through Michael Rutter. He taught me and several generations of students about fundamental issues of normal and abnormal development. His thinking shaped the concept of autism and spread awareness. Rutter's contributions to autism research are extraordinarily wide and far-reaching, but two are particularly noteworthy: he established instruments for diagnostic assessment now used worldwide. He also conducted the first studies on the genetic basis of autism.

Lorna Wing was another of my mentors. As a mother of an autistic daughter she had intimate knowledge of autism. I could not hear enough about her experience and her then very revolutionary ideas about the disorder. Through her studies of a whole population of handicapped children she had realized that there are three critical impairments—the 'triad' of impairments in socialization, communication, and imagination—that hold over a whole spectrum of autistic disorders. At the same time she became aware that social impairment comes in different varieties—the aloof, the passive, and the odd. She was also one of the first researchers to write about Asperger syndrome.

The experimental work of Beate Hermelin (1919–2006) and Neil O'Connor (1918–97) was the foundation of the psychological work that I will report in this book. Their ultimate aim was to link behaviour to the brain, and therefore they adapted the methods of neuropsychology for the study of children. They established a method to study impairments in cognitive abilities, such as language, perception, and memory. One of their innovations was to 'match' a clinical group with another group by equating them in terms of their performance on one test, and then contrasting them on another test. They realized that differences are only interesting if you can relate them to expected similarities. For example, they found that autistic children who remembered jumbled up words as well as other children did worse than other children when remembering whole sentences. This proved an important clue to unlocking the enigma of their minds.

Apart from these professional mentors, I have always learned a great deal from parents of autistic children. The earliest biographical account that I read was by Clara Claiborne Park. It was a revelation. Parents are the real heroes in the history of autism. They made the difference for their children in fighting for services and in promoting research. My personal heroine is Margaret Dewey, the mother of a highly talented autistic son, with whom I have corresponded for decades. She generously told me of the difficulties as well as the triumphs in Jack's life. Her examples, questions, and criticisms continuously clarified my ideas.

The awareness of autism in the 1960s and 1970s was still very low. It was much enhanced by the presence of a small band of parents who got together in National Associations both in the USA and the UK. In London these parents also helped to set up one of the first schools specializing in education for autistic children. This school was led by a gifted teacher, Sybil Elgar. She carefully observed what each individual child was capable of learning, gave clear and simple instructions, used visual aids, and encouraged physical exercise. I often visited this school. Perhaps its outstanding feature was the calming environment and a highly structured and firm teaching style, tempered by kindness.

The children in this school were pioneers too. They resembled the cases described by Kanner and Asperger in astonishing detail. Many did not talk but had some words or phrases that were copied from the adults around them. All had rather low measured IQ, but at the same time many of them showed remarkable talents. One girl had a beautiful singing voice, one boy painted marvellous pictures, another, who was unable to speak, had an astonishing knowledge of prime numbers. All the children seemed to benefit from sports activities and all took part in musical performances. Nevertheless, it became clear that these children would need support throughout their life.

Urgent practical questions: what to do about the children?

At the time virtually nothing was known about what would happen when the autistic child grew up. Now we know that autistic children become autistic adults. They too need a firm structure and a calming environment. The development of appropriate education for children with autism and mental retardation—who often had quite challenging behaviour—was of the highest priority. Some very controversial ideas were tried out for the first time in the 1960s and have since become commonplace. They were called behaviour therapy and behaviour modification, and they were based on the scientific principles of learning theory. Simply put, desired behaviour is rewarded while undesired behaviour is ignored and the reward is withheld. If such a regime is applied systematically, the desired behaviour increases and the undesired behaviour decreases. The success of these methods in managing some appalling problems, for example self-injury through constant head banging, made them acceptable and even popular.

Ivar Lovaas founded a movement in California where his methods have been gradually developed into what is now known as ABA, or Applied Behavioural Analysis. ABA typically involves intensive one-to-one training sessions. But less intensive variants seem to be just as successful, as are variants that emphasize warm emotional contact with the child. All these variants can produce amazing changes. Behaviour can be reinforced even when it is as yet barely present. For instance, parents described to me how over the course of six weeks their little son gradually learned to speak. At first he only managed to blow softly, then more strongly to extinguish a candle. Soon he was able to make some few whispered sounds. Eventually he broke through into producing a syllable, then a word. This seemed like a miracle to them, but it is an often repeated one.

There are other approaches that are geared to compensation and coping strategies rather than to shaping and changing behaviour. In North Carolina Eric Schopler (1927–2006) created a centre for the assessment and amelioration of behavioural difficulties associated with autism and severe learning disabilities. His approach emphasizes a highly structured timetable and uses pictures in a concrete and at the same time imaginative way. It is known as TEACCH and has spread all over the world. You can see the typical visual aids, depicting a series of activities laid out in a clear timetable in almost all schools for autistic children, but also in centres for autistic adults. The child or adult knows that they can always check their own timetable to know where they are in the course of the day and what to do next. This has an enormously reassuring effect and acts as a vital scaffold to organize work and leisure. Actually, different techniques—both to change behaviour and to adapt to behaviour that can't be changed—go hand in hand.

The many faces of autism

Once upon a time it used to be assumed that autism almost always went together with learning disability, or mental retardation, both terms indicating brain pathology associated with low measured IQ. Recent studies have changed this view. Now the spectrum of autistic conditions fully embraces those who have no intellectual impairment when assessed by standard intelligence tests. At present the diagnosis of autism combined with low intellectual ability is made in about 50 per cent of cases, and in 50 per cent is combined with average or even superior levels of intellectual ability.

Autism compounded by learning difficulties

Severe intellectual impairment is due to severe brain abnormality, and this will almost certainly limit emotional and social abilities as well. This is a general effect. However, there are also specific effects of brain abnormality. In autism just such a specific effect can be seen. Here emotional and social abilities are out of line and well below the rest of cognitive abilities. The case of David illustrates this very well. However, if all abilities are low-ish, then it is almost impossible for one particular ability to stand out as lower still.

Intriguingly, not all children with general learning disability, or mental retardation, have social difficulties. In some cases, notably Williams syndrome, the social interests and abilities are way *ahead* of other abilities. You can feel that there is reciprocal communication. These children initiate social contact and try to keep you engaged. The individual with Williams syndrome, even as a young child, will gaze at others, will spontaneously engage with another person, and try and hold and direct their interest. This is also often the case with children with Down syndrome. Clearly, these disorders have their own characteristic profile of strengths and weaknesses, which is different from autism.

What are autistic children with superimposed intellectual disability like? They still are a mystery, and they present many challenges to their parents and teachers. They tend to be very delayed in speaking and may never speak at all. They often appear to be locked into repetitive behaviours, such as rocking, and into routines that are difficult to break. They are more likely to suffer from additional neurological disease, in particular epilepsy. They are also likely to be less attractive in appearance, and they may well exhibit highly unattractive behaviours. The ingenuity of parents and teachers is stretched to the utmost. Such children become adults that can remain difficult to care for. Sadly they are often neglected when people talk about autistic conditions. Most people like to think of autism in high-functioning, not low-functioning, cases. But this is the sharp end of autism. Research is desperately needed to find out what exactly is wrong in the brains of these individuals, and how to improve their lives.

The term high-functioning autism was coined to distinguish it from the previously more familiar cases of mute and withdrawn children. High-functioning children have great possibilities for compensatory learning. Their intellectual resources allow them to develop alternative means to learn social skills. They may carefully observe the social rules, but still not become integrated into the complex social world. They can do well in academic subjects as long as they are taught in ways that take into account their particular strengths and interests. However, the core features of their autism are not necessarily of a milder form. A superior level of intelligence makes a big difference to the vocational achievements that can be attained, but sadly does not make a big difference to the ability to live independently. Many able individuals struggle to cope with even simple demands of everyday life.

Classic autism

When Kanner first described autism, he portrayed a type of child who is now a minority in the autism spectrum. Yet he identified a particular constellation of the signs and symptoms that every clinician recognizes. These children are aloof. If they speak at all, they tend to use rote-learned phrases and words. They do not just show simple repetitive movements, for instance flapping hands and rocking. They show rather more elaborate rituals. They develop complex routines and repeat them faithfully. More intriguing still are their special talents, for instance an exceedingly good memory.

An integral part of this classically autistic child is that it is a child—at the time Kanner described it, virtually nothing was known about their life as adults. Such a child is an icon. It is a beautiful and remote child. The impression of high intelligence can be strong, as is the impression that a normal child is locked inside. But, alas, this is an illusion. It fades as the autistic child grows up.

The autistic child grows up

Child development holds many surprises. A child can grow out of problems. A slow developer might catch up later. But more often than not children with problems become adults with problems. Slow development spotted in childhood may often turn out to be a lifelong learning disability.

The film *Rainman*, first shown in 1989, has had an enormous impact on the general awareness of autism. The main character portrayed by Dustin Hoffman is based on a combination of real individuals with autism. Many of his features were based on Kim Peek, who has become famous as the 'human Google' because of his prodigious memory. For the first time an adult with autism was the centre of attention. Previously only professionals who specialized in children, that is, child psychiatrists, child psychologists, speech therapists, and special educators—but only a minority of all these—knew about the disorder and were able to diagnose it. Neurologists, psychiatrists, and psychologists who worked mainly with adults remained ignorant of the condition at that time. It took a while to face the frightening thought that there were many adults in institutions for the mentally ill or mentally disabled who had not been recognized as autistic.

Dustin Hoffman closely observed real-life cases of autistic adults in his methodical preparation for the movie and modelled himself on them. The autistic man he portrayed was very strange, but also lovable. He looked and acted mentally disabled, and yet had the most amazing skills. He was extremely naive and had no idea that his scheming brother, portrayed by Tom Cruise, wanted to deceive and defraud him. Yet he was able to remember all the addresses in a phone book as soon as he read them and was able to win at a card game in Las Vegas precisely through his amazing memory. Most endearing was the hero's total unselfconsciousness. He did not know how unusual his abilities were. He did not consider how awkward and difficult his rigid behaviour routines were for others, and he unquestioningly accepted the harsh treatment meted out to him by others. This was a new image of autism, one that had not been brought to the public's notice, and it instantly won sympathy.

Rainman is an ambassador of autism. But not all individuals with ASD are lovable eccentrics with amazing gifts. Far from it. Many are very difficult to live with and many have additional problems. It needs to be spelled out that only 10 per cent of individuals with ASD have a truly astounding gift. The families of the other 90 per cent are rightly annoyed when strangers expect that they have a genius in their midst. However, it also needs to be pointed out that among these 90 per cent there are many who have talents that are unusual and remarkable, even if they cannot be described as astounding.

The realistic view about growing up with an autism spectrum condition is provided in a number of biographical accounts. What do they say about the autistic teenager? In many ways he or she is unaware of what it means to be a teenager. They do not have the usual obsession with looking like everyone else in their peer group and wanting to have the same clothes and gadgets. The autistic teenager retains many features that others view as childish. Yet they have the normal sexual urges. Some gain a glimmer of

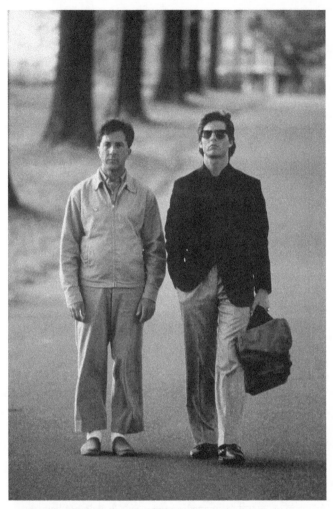

2a. Dustin Hoffman and Tom Cruise starring as two brothers in the film 'Rainman' (1989). This film raised awareness of the adult with autism and exceptional talents (savant syndrome)

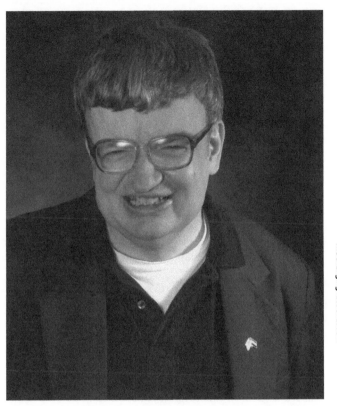

2b. Kim Peek inspired Dustin Hoffman' portrayal of 'Rainman'. Peek reads a whole book in an hour and remembers the text verbatim. He has been described as a walking Google

awareness that they are different. They stick out compared to their peer group. Perhaps they don't care about how they appear to others, and this may be why they now begin to look more handicapped. Now you notice the ungainly gait, the lack of facial expressions. Of course, in a sad way, this is helpful because it is an obvious signal to others that there is a problem.

Increased adaptation

First-hand accounts give a fascinating glimpse into the world of autism. There are an ever increasing number to be found in the catalogues of specialist publishers such as Jessica Kingsley and on websites. These accounts show that many difficulties can be conquered. Compensatory learning can lead to sometimes highly successful lives, including in some cases marriage and children. This is heartening, given that the basic problems in social insight never quite go away. According to these authors they have to be worked on continuously.

One of the most famous autistic writers is Temple Grandin, who has written many books about her own life and can look back on her experiences of over fifty years. Here is a quote from her book *Thinking in Pictures* (expanded edition Vintage Press, 2006, also published on Temple Grandin's website, easily found on Google):

> More knowledge makes me act more normal. Many people have commented to me that I act much less autistic now than I did ten years ago.... My mind works just like an Internet search engine that has been set to access only images. The more pictures I have stored in the Internet inside my brain the more templates I have of how to act in a new situation.

This self-assessment chimes in with what a man with ASD told me recently: 'There are more and more situations I just recognize and don't have to think about.'

One of the big gaps in our knowledge is that we know hardly anything about what happens to people with autism in old age. Do they have the same life span as everyone else? People with intellectual disability—whether autistic or not—usually have a shorter life span, but this could be for a large number of reasons. Sadly, one of the reasons is that they may not alert others to health problems that might be treatable. Furthermore, their repetitive behaviour may include harmful actions, for instance, drinking excessive amounts of water. On the other hand, everyone's life gets more repetitive and restricted as they get older. Many old people see their partners and friends die before them and they have to get used to being lonely, a very hard adaptation for most of us. Is it easier if you never had any friends?

Asperger syndrome

Asperger syndrome has gained such popularity that we need to give it some special attention. It can be seen as a variety of autism with similar biological causes and similar effects on the development of brain and mind, but with somewhat different behavioural manifestations. At least this is what we assume at present.

Asperger syndrome is usually considered a mild form of autism. But this may be deceptive. It may be a form of relatively pure autism where massive learning and compensation are covering up the core problems. There are good reasons for suspecting compensation and covering up. Asperger syndrome goes with high intelligence. Further, the writings of people with Asperger syndrome tell us about their difficulties and how they cope with them. These difficulties seem highly reminiscent of those of people with autism.

Perhaps the strangest fact about Asperger syndrome is that it is not usually diagnosed at all until the age of 8 or even later, sometimes only in adulthood. This is strange, because it is a developmental disorder. It does not start suddenly, but it was always there as family and sufferers almost unanimously proclaim.

Research still needs to uncover the early signs of Asperger syndrome. In contrast to autism language is not delayed, but rather it is often advanced, as in the case of Edward. Further, classic autism implies aloofness, while this is not necessarily found in Asperger syndrome. Individuals with Asperger syndrome often have a strong interest in other people. Children typically seek out adults as valued listeners to monologues, as answerers of questions, and providers of useful information.

A striking difference between autism and Asperger syndrome in childhood is that the child with Asperger syndrome displays high verbal intelligence. This is rightly a source of pride and joy to parents, but might make them overlook a lack of truly reciprocal social behaviour. Again this is illustrated in the case of Edward. As the case of Gary shows, the label is sometimes also applied to individuals with distinct social impairment who also have a mild degree of intellectual impairment. Here, Asperger syndrome is used to indicate an atypical form of autism.

What is the connection to Hans Asperger? Hans Asperger emphasized that autistic disorders appear in many different shades and varieties, including some milder varieties, and including those with high intelligence. He was one of the first people to identify and describe autism not only in children but also in adults. He labelled his cases 'autistic psychopaths' to indicate that the condition was not a disease, but part and parcel of someone's personal make-up. Asperger did not define what we today call Asperger syndrome. Nevertheless it seems fitting that the syndrome is named in his honour.

How did Asperger syndrome get its now well-established place? There are many reasons, but probably the most important was the need to widen the boundaries of the initially narrow concept of classic autism. In the 1980s a number of clinicians began to use the label Asperger syndrome. Lorna Wing in London used it to draw attention to the fact that some people with autistic disorders were highly verbal and even had some social interests. Christopher Gillberg in Gothenburg drew up diagnostic criteria to capture this particular type of individual. This allowed clinicians in other centres to identify similar cases. The criteria that are now generally used for Asperger syndrome are very similar to what in the past was considered a residual or atypical form of autism. They are in almost every respect the same as those for autism. Critically, there is no language delay, and language is often a particular cognitive strength.

Many clinicians took up the label Asperger syndrome with an eagerness that suggested that there was a real need for the category. They saw plenty of individuals who fitted the criteria. These children and adults were on the whole not so severely affected and promised hope of a better prognosis. Not surprisingly, many parents craved the diagnosis Asperger syndrome rather than autism. The popularity of the label rose inexorably.

Rightly or wrongly, Asperger syndrome has become a magnet that attracts cases. One of its attractions is that it has acquired the cachet of being linked to genius. No wonder then that a diagnosis of Asperger syndrome suggests a more interesting and possibly more tractable difficulty than autism. But this is not correct. The difficulty is just as persistent as in other autistic disorders. Nevertheless, Asperger syndrome has a special place in the popular imagination.

A vivid picture of a boy with Asperger syndrome is given in Mark Haddon's book, *The Curious Incident of the Dog in the Night-time*. This book has sold 2 million copies and has been translated into thirty-six languages. It has undoubtedly increased awareness of Asperger syndrome. Chapter 2 starts with the terse description: 'My name is Christopher John Francis Boone. I know all the countries of the world and their capital cities and every prime number up to 7,507.'

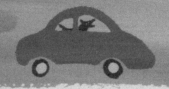

MARK HADDON

THE CURIOUS
INCIDENT
OF THE DOG
IN THE NIGHT-TIME

WINNER
WHITBREAD BOOK OF THE YEAR

3. Book cover of *The Curious Incident of the Dog in the Night-time*

Straightaway we are made aware of the special interests of the boy and his prodigious memory. He claims an affinity to Sherlock Holmes, because he too is super-analytical and, furthermore, he might also be on the autism spectrum.

There are many details in the story that could have been taken from real life and therefore supply telling examples of the typical features of someone who has Asperger syndrome. For example, Chris, who tells the story himself, states that he finds people confusing, that he does not tell lies, that he does not like proper novels because they are lies. He does not understand the purpose of polite language. So he can say 'All the other children at my school are stupid. Except I'm not meant to call them stupid, even though this is what they are. I'm meant to say that they have learning difficulties or that they have special needs.'

Another chapter in the history of autism

Even though it is extremely popular, the label Asperger syndrome is problematic. It is hard to know whether Asperger syndrome will eventually split off and form its own distinct category of developmental disorder. Is it indeed a form of autism and with the same genetic causes as autism? Or is it merely a personality type and not a disorder?

There are now a number of people who have diagnosed themselves as having Asperger syndrome. These individuals often call themselves Aspies, and they feel different from NTs or neurotypicals. They do not need the attention of a clinician. They are perfectly adapted in their everyday lives, occupying a niche that is just right for their special interests and skills. It is not surprising that these people argue that Asperger syndrome is not a disorder. To them it is merely a difference, and a difference to be proud of.

Some campaigners go even further and say that for the whole of the autism spectrum it is wrong to talk of brain abnormalities, wrong to focus on deficits in the mind, and wrong to highlight impairments in behaviour. Instead there should only be talk of differences in brain and mental make-up, some of which represent the autistic mind. This is a strange proposition. To someone who is familiar with classic cases and other severe cases of autism, and knows of the suffering that is associated with autism, it seems perverse. You may disagree, but then this book is not for you.

Chapter 3
A huge increase in cases

Will there be more and more people with ASD?

The one thing that frightened Diane when she was worried about baby Mickey was that she felt bombarded with reports of a huge increase in cases of autism. There was talk of an epidemic.

The stark facts as presented on the website of the Autism Society of America state that since the 1990s there has been an increase of 172 per cent of cases diagnosed as autistic. Actually, it is inevitable that there is a huge increase in recorded cases. Consider that autism was recognized only seventy years ago and became widely known only about twenty years ago. Clearly children and adults are now diagnosed with autism when they would not have been diagnosed before. Ever greater awareness of autism goes hand in hand with the discovery of more and more cases. In earlier times many of these cases would have been classified as mentally retarded.

The extent of this change was revealed in a Californian study. The decrease in mental retardation in Figure 4 corresponds very well to the increase in cases of autism. One might therefore be tempted to say that all that happened is a relabelling. However, there are also other factors at play.

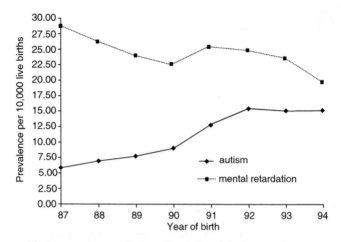

4. The increase in cases diagnosed autistic and the decrease in cases diagnosed mentally retarded in California

Croen, L.A., Grether, J.K., Hoogstrate J. and Selvin, S. (2002) The changing prevalence of autism in California. *Journal of Autism and Developmental Disorders*, 32, 207–15

One factor has to do with the widening of the diagnostic criteria to include milder cases of autism, and cases with normal and high intelligence. These cases would previously not have been diagnosed at all. If they were noticed, they would have been considered eccentrics or loners. This increase is seen in Figure 5, based on the same Californian study.

Widening the criteria

When the question was first asked how common autism is, very narrow criteria were used to identify only the most classic cases. These criteria were social aloofness, elaborate rituals, and insistence on sameness. They turned out to be too restrictive. They apply only to a small subset of children with ASD, and are observed only at a particular stage of their development, mostly between 3 and 5 years. A withdrawn child on getting older often becomes socially interested, and the reverse is also found.

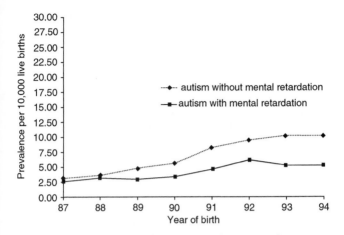

5. Cases without mental retardation increased even more than cases with retardation among those diagnosed with autism in California

Croen, L.A., Grether, J.K., Hoogstrate J. and Selvin, S. (2002) The changing prevalence of autism in California. *Journal of Autism and Developmental Disorders*, 32, 207–15

Likewise, elaborate routines and insistence on sameness can wax and wane over time.

When the behavioural changes over the course of the disorder became evident, and when the extent of individual variation was realized, the use of narrow and specific criteria was abandoned. The criteria were widened towards what is now known as the autistic spectrum. This spectrum includes very typical cases but also rather atypical ones. Young children as well as adults can now be identified, as can individuals of all levels of intelligence. Further, there are mild cases and severe cases. All this adds up to more cases.

What are the numbers now?

The most reliable information to date comes from a British study of 57,000 children aged 9 to 10 years. In this group the total prevalence of cases of autism spectrum disorder was just over 1 per cent. If you only looked at autism cases, then the estimate was 0.4 per cent, with 0.2 per cent fulfilling the narrow criteria of classic autism. Other forms of autistic disorder, including Asperger syndrome, make up around 0.7 per cent.

If we take the 1 per cent estimate seriously, then in the USA, with a population of 280 million, there are a staggering two to three million individuals who have some form of autism; in the UK, with a population of about 60 million, there are at least half a million. Assuming that about 1 per cent of the general population have an autism spectrum disorder, you are almost certain to know someone who is affected. This makes autism as common a mental disorder as schizophrenia or bipolar disorder. But unlike schizophrenia and bipolar disorder, autism is present from early childhood and persists throughout life.

If there was a 'real' increase—what could cause it?

These are scary numbers. Fifty years ago few people were aware of autism. Only the most classic form of autism was diagnosed, and everyone believed this was a very rare disorder. Now, it turns out that there are five times as many classic cases as were estimated then. Is this cause for alarm? Not necessarily. In fact, quite the opposite, if we think of the increase as an effect of increased awareness. Even classic cases had been missed previously. After all, most professionals were ignorant of childhood autism, and institutions for individuals with mental retardation housed considerable numbers of cases, who are now recognized as autistic. I certainly saw such children in special hospitals in the 1960s. Now there are numerous diagnostic centres, and there is a greater availability of services for identified children. All these factors play a part in the huge increase in cases.

Is this all there is to it? How would we know? The awareness of the condition increased gradually. So, we would expect that the

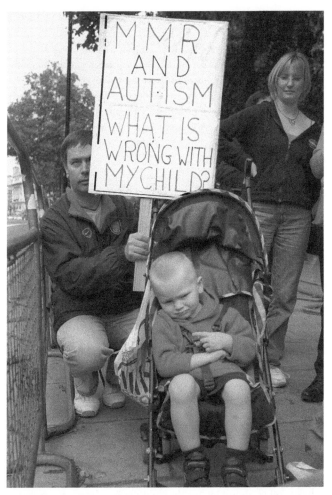

6. A demonstration of parents concerned about a link between autism and MMR

increase in cases is also gradual. We would also expect that there is a levelling off by now.

In fact the increase has been gradual and it has been levelling off recently. Nevertheless, it would be wrong to feel complacent. Parents want to know *all* the reasons for the fast and recent rise in cases of autism spectrum disorders. After all, one other reason could be a new and as yet unknown toxin or virus that is affecting brain development even before birth. If so, it would be incredibly important to find out.

It is very unlikely that autism is caused by some adverse environmental event after birth. As we will see in the next chapter the abnormalities that can be detected in the nerve cells of autistic brains date from well before birth. Nevertheless the personal experience of many parents goes against this. Remember, that many parents reported that their children seemed perfectly normal to them as babies. They had no cause for concern until their child inexplicably changed. This was sometime in the second year of life. They lost the language they already had and completely lost interest in other people.

Scare stories

What sort of unusual and possibly traumatic events happen in the second year that might cause this problem? Vaccination! Vaccination always has an aura of suspicion. By its very nature vaccination is an assault on the small and vulnerable body of a young child. In order to prevent disease, the vaccine provokes a mild form of the disease. These symptoms are temporary and soon shaken off by almost all healthy children. But there are rare cases where things can go wrong, and very wrong, where consequences might even result in brain damage. Now, if vaccinations were multiplied, would the risk be even higher? Precisely such a multiplication was introduced relatively recently. In many countries it became health policy to protect the population with a *single* vaccination against three killer diseases, measles, mumps, and rubella—MMR, the triple vaccination.

Could the triple vaccination be linked to the increase in autism? This hypothesis was clear, plausible, and definitely worth pursuing. And it was pursued vigorously in a number of studies worldwide. Almost unanimously these studies came up with a resoundingly negative answer. Study after study demonstrated that the increase in autism started long before triple vaccination was introduced. The introduction of the vaccine did not go together with a steep rise in cases. The last nail in the coffin was that the withdrawal of MMR in Japan did nothing to stop the rise of cases of ASD. In short, this vaccination is not responsible for increases in cases of autism.

Experts delved into medical records of individual cases, and found that in many there was concern about the child's development already before the vaccination. Even though the negative results were reported in the press, remaining doubts and dissenting views continued to be presented. Indeed the general concern with vaccination has still not disappeared. Are governments and big pharmaceutical corporations out to suppress the truth and deny responsibility? Does the individual ever get a hearing against a powerful corporate defence? On the other hand, do lawyers unscrupulously take advantage of suspicion to make claims for compensation? There have been precedents for both cover-ups and greed. Given previous scandals where public reassurance had been wrong, politicians feel understandably ambivalent and are torn between whether to side with scientists or parental pressure groups.

But it was not only the triple vaccination that worried people. Thimerosal, a derivative of mercury, has been used from the 1930s as an effective preservative for vaccines and for other medicines too until very recently. It has been phased out from 1999. Mercury is a heavy metal, and hazardous because the brain is susceptible to poisoning by heavy metals. It seemed possible that this could be a contributory cause of autism. This is another idea that was worth pursuing. It was taken very seriously by scientists in the USA and particularly in Japan, where in the recent past a terrible environmental disaster due to metal poisoning had occurred. However, researchers were able to rule out mercury poisoning as a cause of autism, comparing children exposed to mercury with those who were not. Furthermore, the number of autism cases continued to increase in California after Thimerosal was removed from vaccines. Nevertheless, the idea still lingers on, and many websites are devoted to this case, including those that offer treatments to remove traces of heavy metals from the body, which are themselves hazardous.

Just as in the case of the triple vaccine, some campaigners are so convinced of their claims regarding Thimerosal that they cannot change their belief. They do not see the relevance of scientific studies that refute the claims. This suggests that other as yet unknown scares could start at any time and take over the lives of campaigners.

Of course there will be more ideas about which environmental factors might contribute to autism. But these ideas need to be anchored in basic research, and basic research has not yet thrown up a credible candidate. On the other hand, blue-sky ideas about possible factors, not anchored in basic research, can waste an awful lot of time and energy.

More reasons for further increases in numbers

Here we take a brief look at the now often blurred boundaries of autistic spectrum disorders.

Diane's colleague at the lab where she worked had a little son who was 7 years old and increasingly difficult to handle. He was constantly doing things he should not do; he had tantrums almost daily; he was aggressive to other children and seemed unable to take part in group activities at school. Moira was at the end of her tether and finally went to a clinic specializing in autistic disorders. Diane was not surprised when Moira announced that Ben had an autism spectrum disorder. The diagnosis brought considerable relief to Moira. Ben was not simply a naughty child, who misbehaved all the time. Instead he just couldn't help being different. Further, she now might obtain special educational resources that she could not otherwise have claimed. But would another professional have diagnosed Ben as having conduct disorder with attention deficit disorder? Quite possibly.

What about the very bright children who are puzzling because, compared to their high intelligence, their social interaction and communication is relatively backward? There may now sometimes be pressure for a diagnosis of Asperger syndrome, when in previous times no one would have worried. In past times these children would have been treasured for their high abilities, and their social awkwardness would have been excused. In today's culture social abilities are arguably more vital to success than ever before, and therefore treasured more highly than ever before.

Perhaps today social incompetence is apparent more often because the demands on social competence are so high. Maybe our social life has become more complicated as people travel more, migrate more, and change jobs more often. If so, it would not be surprising if more children and adults fall short of high demands on social skills. This would include individuals with no particular problems of any kind, but a propensity to be loners and unconventional in their interests. Possibly such people would now be considered for diagnosis, even though they would not have been a generation ago.

We also should consider children with mental retardation of unknown causes. Here social competence is often in line with other abilities and all abilities are very limited. If looked at in detail, the poor social skills turn out not to be the same as in autism, but superficially there might be little difference. However, these children too tend to be increasingly subsumed under the autism spectrum.

I have mentioned these examples because the blurring of the boundaries brings the danger of diluting the concept of autism. This would be a pity, because research has succeeded in identifying the core social features of autism, and has provided methods to differentiate different kinds of social impairment. These are likely to have a different basis in the mind/brain. I have already touched on the characteristic impairment in autism as concerning truly reciprocal interaction.

The widening of the criteria for autistic disorder is a commonly acknowledged reason why there are so many cases today. Is this a good thing or a bad thing? The answer will depend on your point of view. Is there a limit to widening the concept of autism and the stretching of criteria? Does the spectrum really have sharp cut-off points where we can diagnose a person who is affected by autism and a person who is not?

What about the relatives of people with ASD? Are they 'on the spectrum' themselves? Sometimes quite strong and sometimes very watered down symptoms can be seen in the relatives. The observation of very mild autistic features in relatives is greater than might be expected by chance. This has given rise to the idea that there is indeed a broader phenotype of autistic disorders. This means that the genes that are responsible for this phenotype might exist in quite a large number of people, hardly any of whom are autistic themselves. Perhaps these genes predispose them to have children with ASD. This idea is plausible, but as yet speculative.

Are we all—or at least all men—a little bit autistic?

Diane can easily spot people with poor social and emotional intelligence, and most of them seem to be male. In her husband she can spot a sad lack of interest in romantic movies compared to his obsessive interest in football. He seems to spend endless hours going through websites to identify the latest technical gizmos and accessories for his camera. Does this have anything to do with the autism spectrum?

I can see the mocking humour in describing your nearest and dearest or the person next door as 'definitely on the spectrum' or 'a little bit autistic'. It conveys quite a lot of information about the person. But for me this has nothing to do with the true autism spectrum. We are usually talking of a highly educated male who can focus single-mindedly on a particular goal to the detriment of his concern for other people. This male can be an outstanding scientist or artist who doesn't seem to care what others think of him. Sometimes he is a scholar who is not particularly creative, but has the ability to acquire and retain masses of information. He will generally dislike novelty and often rigidly hold to his own opinion.

Being a 'little bit autistic' can be something of a fashion statement. It can also be a welcome excuse for people who are particularly obsessed with their own interests, and don't wish to consider another person's point of view. It can also be a great compliment. It vaguely alludes to genius. Hans Asperger himself implied that a dash of autism was part and parcel of being a creative scientist. He drew parallels between autism, scientific originality, and introversion.

Was Asperger right in claiming that the autistic personality is an extreme variant of male intelligence? In his 1944 paper, which I translated (*Autism and Asperger Syndrome* (1991), 85), he says:

> Girls are the better learners. They are more gifted for the concrete and the practical, and for tidy, methodical work. Boys, on the other hand, tend to have a gift for logical ability, abstraction, precise thinking and formulating, and for independent scientific investigation . . . In general abstraction is congenial to male thought

processes, while female thought processes draw more strongly on feelings and instincts. In the autistic person abstraction is so highly developed that the relationship to the concrete, to objects and to people has largely been lost, and as a result the instinctual aspects of adaptation are heavily reduced.

Simon Baron-Cohen in Cambridge has taken this idea further. He proposes that the outstanding fact about stereotypically male intelligence is driven by a need to have systems. He calls it *systemizing*. However, you need *empathizing* to predict the behaviour of other people and to understand their feelings.

Empathizing and systemizing

Here is a fun thing to do. You can take Baron-Cohen's AQ test on the web. You can find it easily on Google. This is a questionnaire and you have to say whether you agree with a particular statement or not. For instance, 'I prefer to do things with others rather than on my own'; 'I prefer to do things the same way over and over again'. Your answers will count towards your total empathizing and systemizing scores. You guessed it: high empathizing scores are typical of women; high systemizing scores are typical of men. Further, high empathizing scores are typical of humanities students, and high systemizing scores are typical of science students. Interestingly, scientists are over-represented among the relatives of individuals with ASD.

People with Asperger syndrome get very high scores on this questionnaire, much higher than most other people. But don't think you can diagnose yourself, your friends, and relatives! As we have seen already, the diagnostic process is a very long and difficult process, and even experienced clinicians can get it wrong sometimes.

The excess of males

Actually, in most developmental disorders more males are affected than females—for example dyslexia, attention deficit disorder, and

Autism

conduct disorder. It is not clear why this is so. It is not clear whether in autism the excess of males needs special explanation over and above this general phenomenon. Nevertheless, the ratio in autism is quite extreme at the more able end of the spectrum, with 8 to 1. At other parts of the spectrum it seems to vary between 2 : 1 and 4 : 1. Taken together, the excess of males and the typically male preference for systemizing might give a clue to the origin of autism. This is what has led Simon Baron Cohen to investigate whether testosterone, the male hormone, could play a role. The jury is still out.

After all—is there a real increase?

Should Diane be worried that more and more autistic children are born now than were before? Actually, she shouldn't be. Yes there has been a huge increase, but there are good reasons for it. The increase is not a mystery and is not a sign of an epidemic. It can be explained by broadening diagnostic criteria, increased awareness, but also better identification and services for affected children. Further, if people now diagnosed with autism do not always show all the signs in their most typical form, who is to say that there are not more hidden cases that will only gradually come to light?

And yet, Diane cannot help asking whether there is not also a hidden real increase. Science cannot at present give an answer, but should be able to do so in the future. The continued careful monitoring of cases will be essential, but so will vigilance about the boundaries of the diagnostic criteria.

Chapter 4
Autism as a neurodevelopmental disorder

Why is autism a neurodevelopmental disorder?

Mental disorders that are ultimately due to genetic causes and present from early childhood are known as neurodevelopmental disorders. Diane wonders what that means. The *neuro* part of this term clearly refers to the brain. Does this mean it is a question of biology or psychology? It is both! When she sees the term neurodevelopment Diane should think mental development, because brain and mind is the same thing looked at from different points of view. The word development should remind her that we are dealing with a dynamic process. Even tiny deviations from the normal path of brain/mind development at the start can have huge consequences later on.

As Diane informs herself about autism many questions spring to her mind. If you have the genetic fault—never mind what genes are involved—would you then become autistic? Not so. This is only true for vary rare genetic disorders, but unlikely to be the case for autistic disorders. Here the gene fault gives a *predisposition* to become autistic, but what actually happens will depend on other factors. Some of these factors might make autism more likely. These are risk factors. For example, being male means there is a higher risk of autism. Others may make it less likely, for example, being female. These are protective factors.

It would be nice if we knew more about protective factors. Could these factors allow you to escape the consequences of a particular genetic predisposition? Remember Sleeping Beauty? She gets a curse from the evil fairy, meaning she will die young from a poisoned spindle, but she gets a reprieve from the good fairy, meaning that instead of dying she will fall asleep. Clearly, the good fairy does not completely cancel out the bad fairy. But it is still better than if only the bad fairy prevails. In this case, the genetic predisposition sets the programme for abnormal brain development. This starts even before birth.

The development of the brain before birth is one of the great wonders of life. All the nerve cells are born in one place and then have to migrate to their final destination. This is so complex that problems in navigation are only too likely. Other problems can occur in forming the cells in the first place. Finally, when all this is done, another danger looms. This is the process of connecting the cells to each other.

However, this danger does not stop with birth. Brain development is by no means finished at birth. Huge sweeps of brain reorganization take place from time to time during the whole course of development. Changes continue to happen so that highly efficient pathways are created to match up to the skills that are most used. These always involve making more efficient connections between cells. This is often called plasticity.

So, the brain changes all the time, just like the mind. It changes as a result of what we learn. It also changes as a result of maturation, much of which is under the control of pre-set biological processes. Evolution has already taken care of the most basic needs to survive and we don't need much learning to breathe and walk. These are automatically set priorities for the brain, and brain functions to do with thinking and complex behaviour are not top priority. Here faults can be tolerated, more or less. Sometimes, development can work around the problem and nobody knows the difference.

Sometimes, it can't, and problems become obvious. No wonder neurodevelopmental disorders are very complex and very difficult to understand.

Why look in the genes?

Diane wonders why genetic causes are so readily accepted, when there must be other possibilities. What about environmental toxins, immune responses, food allergies, viruses, or bacteria? The studies we discussed in the previous chapter showed that the environmental causes investigated to date, such as Thimerosal, are not causes of autism. Other environmental causes, such as a virus that leads to brain inflammation and subsequent brain damage, have also been studied. Indeed some cases have been described where autism resulted as a severe consequence of acute brain disease. However, these are rare causes of autism, and the symptoms that go with this form of autism tend to be rather severe with intellectual impairment going alongside.

For good reasons, the main suspect has long been a fault in the genetic code. Hans Asperger repeatedly stated that one or other of the parents of the children he saw themselves had distinct features of the disorder. However, it was only in the 1970s and 80s that proof was obtained. This proof came from twins. Michael Rutter and Susan Folstein managed to collect twenty-one pairs of twins, at least one of whom had been diagnosed as autistic. Now they could look at these twins and sort them into identical and non-identical pairs. Only the identical pairs share the identical genes, the non-identical pairs share approximately half their genes, in the same way as other siblings. Of course, both kinds of twin share a substantial part of their environment, before birth and as they grow up. If the identical twins were more often both diagnosed as autistic, then this points to a genetic rather than environmental cause. This was indeed found. In 90 per cent of the identical twin pairs, but only in 10 per cent of the non-identical pairs did both children have an autism spectrum condition. This is a remarkable result. Hardly any other mental disorder is so highly genetic.

Now it gets complicated. In almost all the pairs of identical twins, one twin is more severely affected than the other, and in at least one pair one twin was not affected by autism at all. This is not in the least surprising to geneticists. Remember, genes always interact with other factors. So, in any garden, plants from the identical seed do not show identical growth. In some cases, the position in sun or shade, the presence or absence of water, can markedly affect what the plant will look like and how well it will grow, over and above its genetic potential. In the case of human development, we just don't know what exactly plays the role of seed, sun, or water. For this reason the search for autism genes is actually a search for risk factors and protective factors. I have already likened these to the evil fairy and the good fairy in Sleeping Beauty.

In selected cases of autism mutations in small sequences on particular chromosomes have been found. Sometimes the mutations are already present in one or other of the parents. But these mutations have been identified in a small minority of cases only. So what about the rest, the vast majority? Here, multiple genes are most likely to play a role and these are hard to pinpoint.

Currently huge studies with large numbers of families are under way to hunt for the predisposing genes and to find the additional non-genetic factors that might be necessary for autism to result. But, what are these additional risk factors? It seems that all these evil fairies cast their spell early in pregnancy. Certain viral infections of the mother during pregnancy are thought be a risk factor. Rubella is a known example. An as yet unknown effect of a drug might be a risk factor. For example, thalidomide was found not only to affect the physical growth of the foetus, but also the brain in rare cases, and this resulted in autism.

As far as Diane knows, there was never a case of autism or Asperger syndrome in her or her husband's family. But she cannot be reassured, because autism really can occur seemingly out of the blue. Obviously, in other families autistic disorders can be traced down the generations through the intricate pattern of genes.

Why do several disorders often occur together?

There is another question in Diane's mind: autism can be very complex and it looks as if sometimes several disorders might be superimposed on each other in one and the same individual. This was clearly the case with her colleague's son, Ben. When Gary was diagnosed he had symptoms that could have fitted in with a number of different disorders: dyspraxia, mild learning disability, attention deficit disorder, PDD-NOS, or Asperger syndrome. Which of these labels is the most appropriate? Autism spectrum disorder tends to be the category that trumps others. This is partly because the social and communication impairments have the most serious consequences and partly because autism is most likely to attract services. But why are there such cases like Gary?

Cases who fit more than one disorder are not rare among neurodevelopmental disorders. As a basic scientist I have felt the disdain of clinicians, who know that they daily deal with cases that have more than one disorder at the same time. The term 'comorbid', meaning 'illness on top of other illness', is often used. Many professionals who care for children who have neurodevelopmental disorders feel that the diagnosis is irrelevant, but that the different needs of each individual child, whatever they are, are what actually matters. This is eminently sensible in practice. But it is not satisfactory from a scientific point of view. We need to explain why there are both pure cases and comorbid cases.

One explanation is a shrapnel effect of some initial cause, as opposed to a clean bullet. With the clean bullet, only a single brain system would be affected while the rest of the brain is left more or less intact. With the shrapnel effect more systems will be affected at once. One possible initial cause is a failure in brain development, perhaps a failure in cell migration. The failure can be limited, or it can be more general. In the more general case it would also be more severe in its effect and allow fewer means of compensation.

However, there are other explanations. One novel idea, which is still untested, is instability. Imagine that every developing organism comes with a certain degree of stability or instability. The more stable, the better the organism can withstand the dangers that inevitably occur during development. The more unstable the organism, the more likely that it will not be able to do this. Some of these dangers already lie in the formation of the genetic programme right at the beginning, and others are in the developing brain. In theory, the same dangers may have little or no effect in a stable organism, when they have marked effects in an unstable one.

This theory is testable if the inherent stability of an organism can be measured. Apparently it can be, but it has not yet been applied to autistic disorders. Inherently stable organisms can be recognized by having more symmetrical physical features and fewer physical anomalies, and these can be counted up to give a stability value to each individual. The stable individuals can adapt better when some adversity happens during their development. But of course, only up to a point. Autism may strike even a stable organism, but then this might be the only assault that this organism cannot hold out against. The result would be a 'pure' case of autism. With unstable organisms it is likely that several different adversities would affect development, one blow after the other. The result would be a combination of neurodevelopmental disorders. In the case of Gary for instance, one would expect a number of physical anomalies and fewer symmetrical features of his body, while the opposite would be predicted for Edward. I have

Autism as a neurodevelopmental disorder

to add that this idea is very speculative and there is no evidence as yet to say that it can apply to autism.

The brain in autism

Surely, a condition that has a profound effect on an individual's mind must leave a footprint in the brain. But where to look for this footprint? Indeed, lots of studies exist that have found abnormalities in the brain of people with autism. But what kind of abnormality? There are no holes in the head of autistic people, no tumours, no scars.

The brain consists of millions of neurons and connecting fibres. Are there abnormalities in these neurons, in their individual structure and function? Is this visible via a microscope? Should the footprint of autism also be sought in the living brain at the level of brain systems? Such systems spring into action when we perform particular actions, and think particular thoughts. Here no microscope can help, but the activity of the systems can be made visible by brain scanners. They capture images of blood flowing towards those regions that are particularly active.

Both these techniques have been used and both have yielded information. The autistic brain shows abnormalities in the detailed structure of nerve cells as well as in the structure and level of activity of systems in the living brain. But to interpret these abnormalities is not easy. In fact, we don't yet have enough information and we do not yet know how to put the information from the two sources together.

Under the microscope

Studying brain cells under a microscope, in very fine detail, is painstaking work and done rather rarely. Researchers have found that certain parts of the autistic brain have cells with an abnormal structure. For example, there is a certain type of cell which has a particularly beautiful tree-like structure, and is called the Purkinje cell. These cells are smaller and there are fewer of them in autistic brains, in particular the cerebellum. Likewise, in other parts of the brain, for instance, the limbic system, cells seem to be packed less densely. Cells in the frontal cortex, which are packed together in minicolumns, are smaller and more isolated from each other.

All these facts are still unexplained. However, an important conclusion can be drawn already. The type of abnormalities that are found in the cells themselves suggest that they started early on in foetal development. They are not 'acquired' in later development.

In the scanner

Diane volunteered to be a subject in a brain scanning experiment. She saw a picture of her own brain, looking like an X-ray photograph. Would an autistic brain look different? At first glance the brain of an individual with autism looks fine. At second glance, however, there are plenty of differences. Some regions have been found to be smaller than normal and others larger. Abnormalities have been found in white matter where all the connecting fibres are that link brain regions together. Long-range connecting fibres in particular have been found to be more sparse in autism.

The most important use of scanners is in cleverly designed experiments where it is possible to see the pattern of activity during thinking, imagining, and so on. When Diane was lying in the scanner she was shown a series of pictures. The researcher explained to her that her brain is active all the time, but when she saw nasty pictures compared to nice ones, the amygdala region of her brain burst into extra activity. This was the case even when the nasty picture was flashed up so briefly that she was not even aware of what it was.

So far only a small number of neuroimaging experiments have been done with autistic people. This is because they are difficult to do. One of the main problems is that the person in the scanner must remain completely still. They must not move their head, not even by one millimetre. Also, the scanner is very noisy and dark, and the whole procedure can make people anxious. However, the main stumbling block is with the design of the experiments. Well-controlled designs are unfortunately rare.

For example, we could ask Edward and Gary to say what emotion a person in a photograph displays. This is something that they both find hard to do. But what exactly is it that they find hard in this deceptively simple task? If you think about the task, and cut it down into components, then you can separate out different requirements. For example, to what extent is memory involved, knowledge of words, visual perception? But this is only scratching the surface. Some of the experiments to date have found differences in brain activity during tasks, which people with ASD perform well, but appear to perform differently, using their brain in a different way. Most experiments report that activity in critical brain regions is reduced in autism. This is the case, for example, when the person in the scanner is shown pictures of faces.

Faint traces of brain activity can also be measured through the skull. The methods that are used to measure this activity are EEG, a technique which measures electrical signals, and MEG, a technique which measures magnetic signals. Such signals are given out by the brain all the time, but it is possible to catch the signals at the exact time when a particular event is perceived. So, one can track in real time how the event is processed in the brain. One can compare the signals between one event and another but only by averaging hundreds of trials because the signal is so weak. To do this, researchers may present the same tone through earphones over and over again, but suddenly they present a different tone. The tiny amount of electrical or magnetic activity that occurs at this surprise is an indicator of how sensitive the brain is to differences in these sounds. EEG and MEG techniques have the great advantage that they can be used fairly easily even with young or impaired children. Abnormal responses in autistic children, for example, when looking at faces, have been found.

We do not yet know the significance of any of these findings, what exactly they tell us about anatomical structure or physiological function. Once we can combine the information from the different techniques to study the brain, we will we know where to look for the footprint of autism. This will take time.

There is no doubt that the autistic brain shows abnormal function in different brain regions, but one has to worry about the inconsistency of the results to date. Researchers currently favour the idea that the source of the abnormalities is in the brain's connectivity. One of the most important features of the brain is the massive amount of connections between different regions. The brain has to do a phenomenal amount of work to integrate information that comes from different systems of the brain. It may well be that the abnormality of brain function in autism means that this work is done less efficiently (Figure 7).

Bigger brains

Only recently has it been proposed that young children with autism may have larger heads than other children. Leo Kanner had noticed this, but this observation had long been ignored. Actually, head size at birth in children with autism is no different from other children. The difference arises later, after the first year of life. Then again, at later ages, measurements to date indicate that head size might decrease again. What does this all mean?

Head size, and presumably brain size is not fixed. It changes during one's lifetime. There are indications that in early childhood brain size increases much more rapidly in autism than in typically developing children. During this phase the difference between the

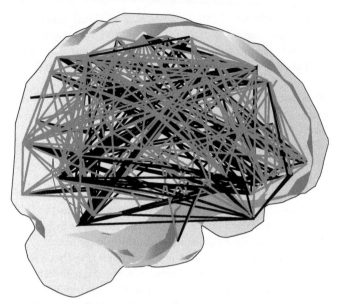

7. There are multitudes of connections between brain regions. It is possible that the brain is connected less well in autism. There could be fewer connections, or misconnections

groups is very large. However, the brain of typically developing children also increases and catches up eventually.

At this point the definitive study following different individuals over time has yet to be done. But we can assume that the young brain waxes and wanes during development. Perhaps in autism there is more waxing than waning, at least during early childhood. What could be behind this bulge in brain size?

Pruning overgrowth in the developing brain

Diane is reminded of her garden, where shrubs proliferate and have to be pruned to be kept from choking themselves. It makes sense that the brain too has phases of overgrowth and pruning. If the number of nerve cells is more or less fixed at birth, then it is

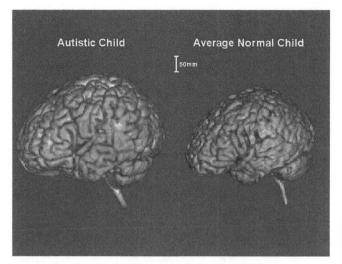

8. Example of a very large brain as shown by some children with autism. Many children with autism have small head size at birth, but show an excessively large increase in head size after the first year of life. From late childhood onwards decreases in headsize have been reported

presumably the connections between nerve cells that get pruned. These connections are quite like plants, and particularly roots of plants, with many branches (called dendrites) that spread out to make connections with other branches from other nerve cells. At the point of contact between these branches, there are most intricate devices, called synapses. These are miniature factories that regulate what goes in and out. This has all been studied in the lab of neurobiologists who can look at just a few brain cells under the microscope. Often these cells come from mice, but they work in exactly the same way in humans.

A good gardener, like Diane, often has to prune bushes, hedges, and trees in her garden. In the case of the brain the role of the gardener is partly taken by the genes that control the process, and partly by learning. Learning is a way of sorting out the necessary connections from the unnecessary ones. We can imagine that in the autistic brain one or both these 'gardeners' are negligent. Perhaps there are too many connections, which result in misconnections.

Unfortunately, no direct evidence exists that could tell us exactly what it is going on. We also need more knowledge about the normal development of the brain. There is a lot of work to do.

Some preliminary conclusions

I cannot hide the fact that there is little specific to report about the causes of autism, nor about the brain in autism. In this chapter I have therefore stuck to more general issues but couldn't resist adding one or two speculations, like instability of the developing organism, and pruning in the developing brain. You can read hundreds of scientific articles and whole books about the biological factors involved in the causation of autism and the medical conditions that accompany autism sometimes. There are also hundreds of studies using structural and functional brain imaging techniques attempting to tell you important facts about the brain in autism. However, soon there will be other papers and books, and they will all tell slightly different stories.

What conclusions can Diane draw from the work in progress? First, there is not just one cause of autism but many. Different mixes of predisposing genes might be implicated in different cases. Brain abnormalities that can be seen under the microscope suggest that they stem from a very early stage in foetal development. Larger brains in autistic children are an interesting new finding, but it is not yet known what this means.

Chapter 5
Social communication: the heart of the matter

What are the problems in social communication and why are they there?

Dare I say that the really interesting facts about autism are not about the brain and not about genes? They are about the mind. I firmly believe that even if we did know everything about the causes of autism, we would still not understand autism. We need to know what it is like to be autistic.

Why can't you fully share in the social world if you are autistic? Is there an extra social sense, beyond sound, sight, or touch, that they don't have? Children born blind or deaf can still receive and respond to social signals, but autistic children cannot do this. From now on we are going to look at insights from psychological research that lead us to the heart of autism. In this chapter we look at three big ideas that a number of scientists have put forward to clarify what autistic failure of social communication is all about.

The first big idea: reading minds

Let's go back to Mark Haddon's novel, *The Curious Incident of the Dog in the Night-time*. Christopher, the hero in the book, can solve difficult logical problems. But he does not get the social signals that are glaringly obvious to everybody else. He does not know who is lying and who is trying to help him. Why does he have these problems? This question, unlike many of our questions so far, has an answer.

> ...one day Julie sat down at a desk next to me and put a tube of Smarties on the desk, and she said, 'Christopher, what do you think is in here?'
>
> And I said, 'Smarties.'
>
> Then she took the top off the Smarties tube and turned it upside down and a little red pencil came out and she laughed and I said, 'it's not Smarties, it's a pencil.'
>
> Then she put the little red pencil back inside the Smarties tube and put the top back on.
>
> Then she said, 'If your Mummy came in now, and we asked her what was inside the Smarties tube, what do you think she would say?' ...
>
> And I said, 'A pencil.'
>
> That was because when I was little I didn't understand about other people having minds. And Julie said to Mother and Father that I would always find this very difficult. But I don't find this difficult now. Because I decided that it was a kind of puzzle, and if something is a puzzle there is always a way of solving it.

The book is only a story, but the experiment that is described here was carried out some twenty years before. That much time is needed for new theories to be tested thoroughly and for a new idea to become widely known. Scientific breakthroughs rarely happen overnight, and are rarely due to a single person. On the contrary, they usually rely on the work of many people over many years.

How do scientists study someone like Christopher? How can they find the reason for his strange problems? If you have read the book, you may remember that Christopher has to use logic to find out what his father, or anyone else, knows and believes. Only a person with autism has to do this. Most of us readers don't use logic. Instead we have an automatic indicator. Think of a SatNav that tells you where you are in relation to space. The brain has a device that tells you where you are in relation to other people. We *just know* that people or characters in a story have wishes, feelings, and beliefs and most of the time we know pretty exactly what they are; most of us are born to read minds. Christopher can't read minds.

The social part of our brain and mind normally allows us to react automatically to other people's behaviour. We don't have to think about it, but we can explain what people do by taking into account what they think and want. This has been dubbed 'mentalizing' or having a 'Theory of Mind'. In autism the mentalizing mechanism has gone wrong.

The first ever test of the big idea is illustrated in Figure 9. It goes like this: Sally has a basket, and Anne has a box. Sally has a marble and puts it inside her basket. Then she goes to play outside. While Sally is away, naughty Anne takes the marble from the basket and puts it into her own box. Now, it is time for Sally to come back. She wants to play with her marble. Where will she look for her marble? Most children by the time they are 5 years old, can answer this question with great confidence. Sally will look for her marble in the basket, because that is where she believes it is. Her belief is now false; we know where the marble really is, but Sally does not know this.

In contrast, even very clever children with autism find the Sally–Anne test very hard. They tend to say that Sally will look where the marble *really* is. They do not take into account Sally's now outdated belief. They will eventually learn what is going on,

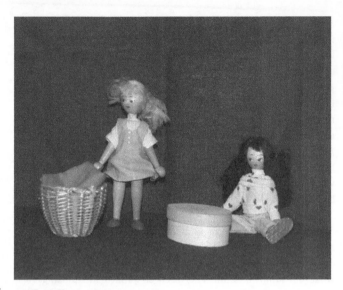

9. The Sally–Anne test

This test was used by Baron-Cohen, S., Leslie, A. and Frith, U. (1985) Does the autistic child have a "theory of mind"? *Cognition*, 21, 37–46

but it takes them much longer than normally developing children, and what they learn is something different from the easy and automatic grasp of the situation. In autism mentalizing never seems to be effortless and automatic. One extremely able person with autism said about his difficulties in social interaction, 'I sit down after an exchange to figure out intentions, beliefs, etc. I definitely need to do this "off-line", after-the-fact, not in real-time.'

So, learning does go on but it often misses the crucial point. For instance, the mother of a young man with autism said: 'I have taught him to apologize when he has hurt somebody's feelings. He always does this—except he doesn't recognize when the feelings are hurt. He is over-doing it.' But there are many cases with far less understanding. One young man was always staring at others because he believed that his thoughts would then be known to the person he was staring at.

The Sally–Anne test is an illustration of an explicit and fully conscious form of mind reading, a form that is mastered relatively late in development. Recent research on the typical development of mentalizing has succeeded in showing evidence for the ability in infants in their second year of life. This evidence is obtained from the eye gaze pattern of young children when they watch a scenario, a bit like the Sally–Anne test. For example, they gaze longer—and show surprise—when Sally looks where the marble really is, and not where she must think it is. So they obviously have a strong expectation of where Sally will look, and are curious about seeing a different outcome. Research in progress indicates that autistic children do not have this capacity for these quite unconscious forms of mind reading. Furthermore, it is doubtful if they ever acquire them. Lack of intuitive mentalizing has been nicknamed mindblindness.

Mentalizing in the brain

The big idea has led to the discovery of a previously unsuspected brain system. This brain system is dedicated to mentalizing. It was discovered with the aid of brain scanners. One challenge was to create stimuli that invite spontaneous mentalizing and contrast them with stimuli that don't do that. The extra brain activity in this comparison tells us which brain areas are involved in mentalizing. These areas are shown in Figure 11.

It turned out that simply showing people animated movies could bring out this contrast. The actors in the movies were two little triangles. In some movies they interacted with each other as in Figure 10, and in other movies, they moved randomly.

Interacting Triangles

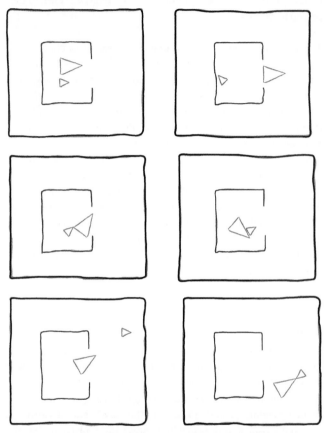

10. Movement can give the illusion that the triangles are creatures interacting with each other. The animated sequence illustrated in the stills above evokes the following interpretation: The big triangle (mother) and the little triangle (child) are in the house. The mother goes outside and gently persuades the initially reluctant child to go out as well. At last the child ventures outside, and both play happily together.

Castelli, F., Happé, F., Frith, U. & Frith, C. (2000) Movement and mind: A functional imaging study of perception and interpretation of complex intentional movement patterns. *NeuroImage*, 12, 314–25

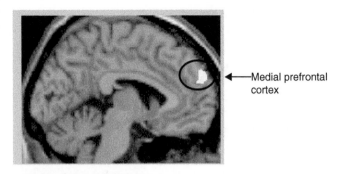

Medial prefrontal cortex

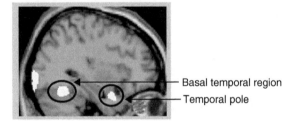

Superior temporal sulcus/ temporal-parietal junction

Basal temporal region

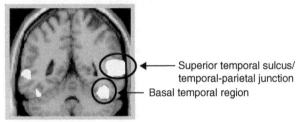

Basal temporal region

Temporal pole

11. Regions of the brain that are active during mentalizing in the normal brain. They show reduced activation in people with autism and have weaker connectivity

Adapted from Castelli, F., Happé, F., Frith, U. & Frith, C. (2000) Movement and mind: A functional imaging study of perception and interpretation of complex intentional movement patterns. *NeuroImage*, 12, 314–25

Problems with the first big idea

The mindblindness idea has been tested vigorously over many years, but there are still loose ends that will have to be tied up in the future. One of the main criticisms is that difficulties in mentalizing are not found in all people on the autism spectrum. Let's assume that this criticism isn't just based on using the Sally–Anne test. After all, this is just one test, and to test mentalizing you need a full battery of tests with stringent controls.

The second criticism of the big idea is that people who are not autistic, but have other disabilities, also fail mentalizing tasks. This criticism is not fatal. You can fail the tasks for different reasons. After all, depending on the task, typically developing children can fail them too. For example, if you use the Sally–Anne task, then children below age 4 fail it, and so do deaf children at much older ages. But in each case there are many other indicators that show that they can mind-read. Another criticism of the big idea is that the social impairment of autism emerges before mentalizing emerges in typical development. Recent research with infants who show the capacity for intuitive mentalizing in their second year of life may answer this criticism.

A fair criticism is that mentalizing failure disregards the emotional aspects of social communication, especially those aspects that allow the automatic and intimate sharing of feelings. These emotional aspects are addressed much better in the second and third of the big ideas.

The second big idea: driven to be social

David never seemed to look at people from when he was a small child. He even seemed to avoid eye contact and turned away when he was held for a hug. He did not mould his body to that of his mother's when she tried to cuddle him. He stiffened when he was picked up. His willingness to look at familiar people increased somewhat as he got older, but still he did not relish physical contact and was happiest when on his own.

This is the second big idea: autistic individuals lack the biologically hard-wired drive to be social. Evidence for this drive is seen straight from birth. The baby prefers to look at faces rather than other objects, and seeks to listen to speech above other noises. But this is only the beginning. In the first year of life the infant is constantly engaged in interaction, primarily with the mother, but also with other people. These interactions are highly pleasurable.

One easy-to-observe example is the sharing of affect, whether smiles or frowns. Experiments have shown that infants are exquisitely sensitive to the timing of face-to-face interaction with their mother. In an experiment mother and baby could see and hear each other via a monitor. They could still interact very happily, showing beautifully synchronized movements and expressions. If the mother's picture on the monitor was frozen for a brief moment, this immediately evoked distress. The healthy young baby is a thoroughly social creature.

Proponents of the second big idea have also claimed joint attention as a sign of the hugely important drive to be interested in other people. Actually, joint attention has equally been claimed by proponents of the first big idea—as a first sign of mentalizing. Both views might be correct.

There must be a brain basis for this precociously established social drive. It is presumably necessary for the survival of young babies. This brain basis may be faulty in autism. A number of autism researchers have independently targeted regions of the brain that are known as the social brain. One particular idea is that there is a brain system underpinning our instinctive emotional responses to others, located predominately in the amygdala. A fault in this system could give rise to a conspicuous class of social and communication problems in autism. These have in common an indifference to other people, difficulties in even looking at people and, as a further consequence, no joint attention and difficulties in recognizing people.

A world of faces, bodies, and eyes

The second big idea makes us aware that we are all living in a world of people. People, with their faces, bodies, eyes, and their history, are not just always around us, but are constantly in our minds, in our memory, our dreams, and our imagination. Is it possible that this is not the case for autistic people? What a very different inner life they would have. When we meet a friend again after some years, we can effortlessly remember whether we parted amicably or had a disagreement. Imagine if you were unable to do this. You would surely think the world of people complicated and unpredictable.

Here is an extract from what an anonymous person with Asperger syndrome wrote:

> Something that most of us find difficult to remember is to whom we have said something and to whom not. Neurotypical people seem to be able to keep a mental file or record for every person they know with minute details, down to the fibs that have been said along with a mental note to keep them in mind.

One of the most important things about the world of people is faces. And in faces it is the eyes that attract our attention.

In an imaginative study scientists tracked the eye gaze of people as they watched the famous Hollywood film *Who's Afraid of Virginia Woolf* with Elizabeth Taylor, George Segal, Sandy Dennis, and Richard Burton in the starring roles. This film, made in 1966, provides a large number of scenes of intense interpersonal interaction. Hence there were plenty of opportunities to observe exactly where you look when you watch such highly meaningful interactions. In fact, most people look at the characters' eyes, often

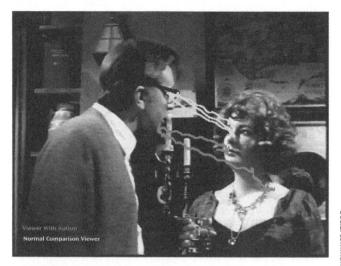

12. People were shown scenes from a film and their eye gaze was recorded. The darker lines indicate the eye gaze of individuals with ASD, the lighter lines that of ordinary individuals. The latter tended to look at the eyes for preference. People with ASD are more likely to look at the mouth

From Klin, A., Jones, W., Schultz, R., Volkmar, F., and Cohen, D. (2002) Quantifying the social phenotype in autism. *American Journal of Psychiatry*, 159, 895–908

switching from one to the other. In contrast, people with Asperger syndrome tended to look at the characters' mouths rather than their eyes. Often they looked at places in the picture that did not contain people at all.

Exciting work is being done on how autistic people respond to the eye gaze of people, when they deliberately look at objects. Normally, we expect to find an object of interest in the place where a person looks, especially if that person looks at us first, signalling the intention to communicate something. If there is no object we feel let down. This effect can clearly be seen in an increase in brain activation in a region at the side of the brain, around the superior temporal sulcus. In autism this increase does not happen. This region of the brain has come up in many neuroimaging studies of autistic brains as deviant. It is a crucial part of the social brain and also plays a part in mentalizing. Figure 10 shows where this region is located. It could well be that the underlying brain areas associated with a social drive and with mentalizing are overlapping. Future research will clarify this.

Problems with the second big idea

It is very likely that there are innate mechanisms in the normally developing brain that prefer social stimuli to any other stimuli. It is likely that these are faulty in autism. However, if autistic children were missing a social drive it should be possible to demonstrate this pretty soon after birth when this drive can normally be seen in strength and abundance. Indeed, according to this big idea, it should be possible to diagnose autism in the first year of life. Yet, as we have seen in Chapter 1, this is difficult to do. In cases of regression one of the key signs is a loss of social interest. Remarkably, parents feel strongly that in early infancy this interest was present.

The third big idea: the human mirror system

The third big idea starts from ground-breaking work with monkeys done by researchers in Parma. 'Monkey see monkey do' is a popular saying, but who would have thought that it encapsulates a basic truth about the brain? The researchers in the Parma group recorded the firing of neurons in a particular brain region. To their own surprise they discovered that there was activity in the exact same cell whether the monkey saw that action being performed by an experimenter, say grasping a peanut, or when he grasped the peanut himself. These brain cells acted as mirrors.

This was a hugely important finding since monkey and human brains are very similar. Even though it is as yet not possible to record the firing of brain cells directly in humans, we can assume that there is a mirror system in the human brain.

When we observe others performing an action our brain's mirror system is automatically active so that we are ready to perform the action ourselves. This is very useful because it allows us to understand other people's actions in a very direct way. When we perform the action, then the same neurons are active as when we observe the action in someone else.

Therefore the mirror system makes an automatic link between seeing and doing, and it is a mechanism that enables us to understand the meaning of the action that another person performs. In other words, as far as the mirror neurons are concerned they don't care whether it is us or another person who performs an action.

But this is not all. The idea of a mirror system goes well beyond action. It is exciting to think that a similar mechanism is responsible for understanding the inner intentions and even the inner feelings of other people. After all, intentions and feelings are usually accompanied by movements in the face and body. Further, does a fault in the mirror system of the brain explain lack of empathy? Empathy is often defined as a way of unconsciously copying the feelings of another person. Could a fault in this mechanism explain many of the social difficulties in autism? This is the third big idea.

There is still little evidence for the third big idea and there are both supporting and negative findings. Here are the negative findings. One prediction is that children with autism would show less good understanding of other people's goals and goal-directed actions. Also their imitation of actions should be poorer. Neither seems to hold under strict experimental conditions.

Figure 13 illustrates the success of an autistic boy in imitating precisely what the experimenter does. Her goal is to point to a particular chip on the table and even rather young children with autism can understand this automatically. They can imitate the

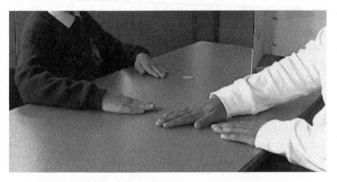

13. Imitation of hand movements. The experimenter pointed to particular chips on the table with either hand. Children were asked to copy this. Children with ASD performed exactly the same as typically developing children. They understood the goal of the experimenter and pointed to the same chip but using their most convenient hand

Based on Hamilton, A.F.d.C., Brindley, R.M., Frith, U. (2007) How valid is the mirror neuron hypothesis for autism? *Neuropsychologia*, 45, 1859–68

pointing action. Like typically developing children they pay more attention to the goal than to the hand that the experimenter used. They tend to use the hand that is nearest to the goal chip, rather than the other hand, even when the experimenter used it herself.

It is a relief to know that autistic children can understand goals, even when they have difficulty in understanding the more complex motivations of people's behaviour. However, this was an example of imitation to order, not spontaneous imitation in a typical social context. In fact, there is something amiss in autistic children's ability to imitate. There is also something amiss with their ability to inhibit imitation. This is seen, for instance, in the tendency to echo speech, a classic feature of autism. A deeper reason for abnormalities in imitation could be to do with mindblindness. Autistic children have difficulty understanding the signals that invite or prohibit imitation in particular communicative contexts.

Emotional resonance

Let's look at the positive findings. The broken mirror theory is particularly attractive when explaining why autism goes together with poor sharing of affect in social situations. People with autism apparently show less activity in the mirror system when they observe other people's facial expressions and gestures. This finding still needs to be replicated in further studies. It would help us to explain the apparent lack of emotional connectedness in autism.

One of the recurrent themes in descriptions of social impairments is the lack of emotional resonance. We all know of the warm glow of feeling in synchrony with another person's feelings. In contrast, apparent indifference to other people's feelings is surely one of the hardest things to bear when you live with an autistic person. Angela, the wife of Andrew, a man with Asperger syndrome, was extremely distressed when her father died. Andrew showed no sympathy and talked loudly and disparagingly about his father-in-law, saying it was his own fault that he had cancer, since he smoked. He never comforted Angela but seemed annoyed that she did not carry on with her usual routine. Ironically, Andrew is very aware of other people's suffering in an abstract sense. He always gives generously to a charity in Africa.

There is clearly a difference between the abstract form of empathy, which Andrew was certainly capable of, and the form of empathy for the feelings of another person as conveyed in body language, and felt as if by contagion. The mirror system seems to provide the mechanism for such a contagion.

One facial movement that is known to be very contagious is yawning. It is not even a feeling, it is a primitive reflex that does not have to be learned. Japanese researchers showed yawning faces in still pictures to children with autism and recorded their tendency to yawn. The results are shown in Figure 14. Autistic

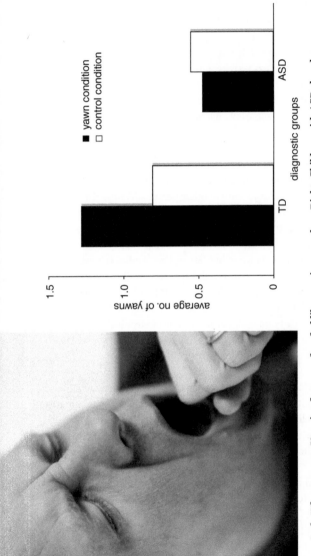

14. **Left:** When we see a Yawning face, we often feel like yawning ourselves. **Right:** Children with ASD show less contagious yawning when looking at yawning faces compared to faces simply opening their mouths than typically developing children (TD)

Adapted from Senju A., Maeda M., Kikuchi Y., Hasegawa T., Tojo and Osanai H. (2007) Absence of contagious yawning in children with autism spectrum disorder. *Biological Letters*, 22, 706–8 children showed far less contagion than normally developing children. This finding will need to be replicated also with adults. Similar experiments are now being carried out with emotions.

Problems with the third idea

The broken mirror theory is still new. It needs to be refined to explain which social interactions go wrong in autism. Like the other big ideas, it cannot explain everything about the impoverished social life that autism entails. However, it offers an exciting possibility: it could help us to understand why in autism there is the curious lack of emotional responsiveness. It is possible that this idea will in the future define a cognitive phenotype that can be matched eventually to a genotype. It is possible to imagine a person exhibiting signs of all three cognitive phenotypes, mentalizing failure, lack of social drive, and mirror system failure. It is also possible to imagine individuals at different places on the autism spectrum, who fit just one of them.

Language and communication

Is this a separate problem in autism? Or is it part and parcel of the social impairment? If so, which of the big ideas would deal best with it?

Imagine the way we interact with a cash machine, and then imagine how we interact with another person. An autistic person would not see much difference between the two situations. This could be due to a lack of social drive, the second big idea.

The first big idea makes a different stab at the problem. Communication is truly reciprocal interaction and this is what mindblindness tries to explain. Reciprocal interaction is more than just asking and answering questions. We always probe how much our conversation partner has understood, how much he or she has been persuaded by us. We would not do this when faced with a machine.

Mindblindness has dire consequences for ordinary two-way communication. For example, people with autism don't see the point in gossip and banter. We normally love this because it allows us to do much more than exchange information. In the way we choose our words, we display our own attitudes to the world. Moreover we learn about others' attitudes towards us. They don't tell us directly, but the SatNav-like device in our brain has a sense for it. In contrast, a person with autism is geared only to the exchange of information itself. So you should not tease them, not make jokes, and not use irony. Their first inclination would be to take all remarks at face value. Note that with normally developing children there is no need to tell them not to take things too literally. They understand this quite by themselves.

It is easy to confuse talking with communicating. When David did not talk, his parents were desperate for him to speak. They felt sure the doors to communication would at last be opened when he began to use words. But, sadly, this did not happen. David now speaks, but he still does not communicate. The doors to communication do not have to wait for language to be unlocked. If they are locked, then language will not be the key. You only wish to communicate if you are aware that what is in your mind is interestingly different from what is in the mind of the other person. This fits with the first big idea, mindblindness. But the other ideas too can explain lack of communication. The second big idea suggests that communication never gets off the ground due to a lack of social motivation; the third, that this is due to a lack of mirroring of another person's feelings, intentions, and even actions. Indeed, we communicate not only by talking to each other, but also by the way we move, our face, our hands, in fact our whole body. We often give away what we feel with our body language what we try to conceal with our words.

Thus, all three big ideas have something to contribute to the explanation of the problems in communication. These are the problems that are at the heart of autism.

There is no blanket social failure

In this chapter we have looked at three different explanations for the cruel and often devastating social and communication failure in autism. But it would be a mistake to believe that people with autism have no social competence at all. In our eagerness to find reasons for the problems, we must not forget the islets of social ability.

Ronald belonged to a club for stick insect enthusiasts. Members compare notes and pictures of stick insects: there are over 1,560 species in the UK. Every street lamp has its own group of stick insects. Ronald hoped to find a girlfriend through the club. There was in fact one girl who was a member, but she was not what he wanted, not being a blonde and not being very pretty. There is nothing wrong with the ability to judge attractiveness of women in most autistic men.

Four-year-old Sebastian was almost totally self-absorbed. And yet, one day his mother observed that he brought a blanket to cover her when she was resting on a sofa. Examples of kindness that transcend the typically strong egocentrism of people with autism spectrum disorders are not common, but they exist. Likewise, examples of empathy exist, even though a lack of empathy is frequently seen as typical of autism. In fact, lack of empathy is common in people with another disorder, psychopathy. Psychopathy is an emotional disorder, where moral judgement is affected. However, unlike people with autism, psychopaths are excellent mind readers and know just how to deceive and defraud other people.

Sylvia is quite oblivious of other people—or so it seems. She does not have much social interest. She also lacks the ability to mentalize. She pays so little attention to people that it is hard to say whether she is aware of emotional expressions and whether she even remembers people's faces.

A big surprise came when she took part in an experiment that investigated knowledge of gender and race stereotypes. She had excellent knowledge these stereotypes! In fact Sylvia was not the only one who surprised us with this knowledge. The other autistic children tested also showed evidence of having the same social stereotypes as typically developing children. For example, the experimenter asked the following question about a picture of a boy and a girl. 'Here is Jack and here is Mandy. One of these children has four dolls. Which one has four dolls?' Sylvia unerringly pointed to the girl.

Besides gender stereotypes (playing with dolls, cooking, caring for others, and so on), racial stereotypes were probed also. While gender stereotypes might conceivably be absorbed by observation, the racial stereotypes could not have been based on direct experience. They are untrue! How could black be associated with being dishonest, dirty, unfriendly and white with being honest, clean, friendly? Sylvia pointed to the picture of a brown coloured person when the experimenter asked: 'Which person has stolen a wallet?' and to the pink coloured person when the experimenter asked: 'Which person has many friends?' Just the same as the other children, whether autistic or not. How did she acquire these stereotypes? Presumably by absorbing implicit cultural attitudes. This means she is not impervious to these attitudes, and this raises the possibility that unexpected types of social learning might be possible for children with autism that have not yet been exploited.

These few examples show that our social world is not completely closed to individuals with autism. What other pockets of our social world are open to autistic people? There might be more surprising answers in future research.

Chapter 6
Seeing the world differently

The savant mystery

Perhaps the most awe-inspiring fact about autism, the fact that all the fictional accounts of autism celebrate, are the savant talents. These talents can flourish even in people who have no language and are severely intellectually impaired. The term comes from *idiots savants*, literally 'the foolish wise ones', and reminds us that originally the talents were noticed in people with very low intellectual abilities and presumably very abnormal brains. Later the term 'savant' came to be used for individuals who, whatever their intellectual ability, have uncommon and unusual talents. The talents are acquired spontaneously and often discovered only accidentally. Kim Peek is able to memorize whole books by just reading them. No one had ever taught him this. I knew a boy who could look at a page of numbers of increasing size and pick out the prime numbers with lightning speed. Other astonishing examples are musical and artistic productions.

Figure 15 shows an example by a deservedly famous savant artist. Stephen Wiltshire has been filmed while drawing the cityscape of Rome, which he saw from a helicopter. You can see this film on the web. Stephen memorized everything he saw in the 45-minute ride and needed three days to draw the full panorama. He drew first not a grand outline of the map and the main features, but he

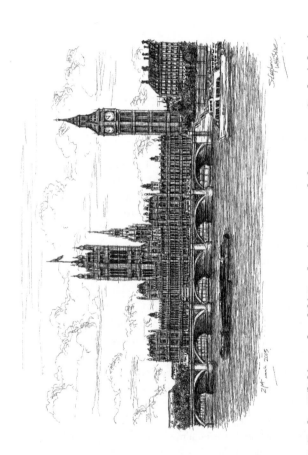

15. Stephen Wiltshire produced this London cityscape purely from memory. Stephen's drawings are highly accurate, but they are also creative and original

started with the detail of St Peter's basilica, in the middle of his drawing. He then proceeded to fill the surface to the right, and then the surface to the left, all in meticulous detail. In this way he created a very accurate picture, as faithfully stored in his memory. How can this extraordinary phenomenon be explained?

Unexpected strengths

Not every autistic child has outstanding talents. However, most have unexpected abilities. I recently found a message by a 46-year-old woman posted on a website for people with ASD: 'I never knew that jigsaw puzzles were supposed to be done using the picture rather than the shapes.' This chimed in with one of the earliest observations I made when studying children with autism: Some of them were able to complete a jigsaw puzzle upside down, without the aid of the picture. This led to one of the first experiments I did. I invited children to do a puzzle with a simple colour picture. Sometimes, the pieces were straight; sometimes they had jagged edges. The autistic children I tested were delighted to fit the jagged pieces together and didn't care about the picture. The non-autistic children were interested in making up the picture and were pleased when they could use the pieces with straight cut edges and did not have to fiddle with the tricky edges.

In my mind the result of this simple experiment fitted together with results of other experiments. In these experiments autistic children had to listen to words, either jumbled up in a meaningless way, or presented as a proper sentence, and then immediately recall them. Most children remembered more when they were presented as a sentence, and could manage even when the sentence was quite long. Not so autistic children. Instead, some of them remembered long random strings of words astonishingly well.

Yet other experiments showed that autistic children were incredibly good at finding hidden shapes embedded in larger meaningful pictures. Some of them love the 'Where is Wally' books and can do better than their siblings. There are plenty of results to show that autistic children perform exceedingly well on some and poorly on other tasks. Here it should be possible to find a clue to their strange intelligence, an intelligence that could appear very high and very low at the same time.

One idea was that autistic children cared for the possibly meaningless elements of a sentence or a picture, but not for the meaning of the whole sentence or the whole picture. If so, this was a completely different way of processing information. Could this processing style also lead to a different kind of intelligence? Could it explain special talents? These questions led to the theory of weak central coherence, the fourth big idea. What this theory tries to explain is illustrated in Figure 16, on the one hand, and by an example from Mark Haddon's book (p. 7), on the other. Here Christopher is clearly not as impressed or frightened by the police turning up as he should be, especially as they are going to take him to the police station. Instead, he notes some minute details about their appearance.

Then the police arrived. I like the police. They have uniforms and numbers and you know what they are meant to be doing. There was a policewoman and a policeman. The policewoman had a little hole in her tights on her left ankle and a red scratch in the middle of the hole. The policeman had a big orange leaf stuck to the bottom of his shoe which was poking out from one side.

Narrow interests and restricted behaviour

Different people with autistic disorder have written about their liking for detail and their ability to focus on detail. A focused interest in detail can appear narrow to others and narrow interests are a key feature for the diagnosis of autism spectrum disorder and particularly Asperger syndrome.

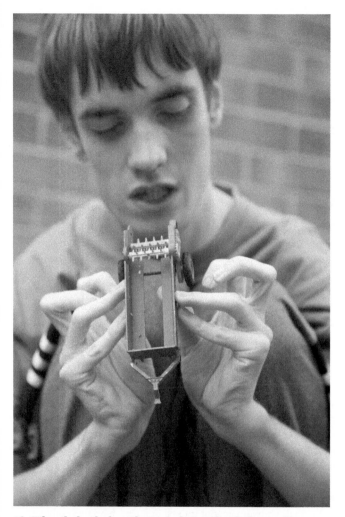

16. When the boy looks at the toy car he sees details that would normally escape us. It is as if these details have precedence over the whole object. Thus, the boy does not play with the car as a car, but is more interested in its parts, especially those that he can flick, turn, and rotate

Charles, who has Asperger syndrome, wrote in an email: 'I have unusually strong, narrow interests. This is the feature that most strongly and obviously applies to me. Between the ages of 11 and 18 I had an interest in maths that was extremely strong indeed. From 4½ to about 13 I was very interested in Rupert Bear. From about 7 to 13 I was very interested in astronomy. In the last few years I have been very interested in learning foreign languages.' Charles is unusually gifted. Characteristically, he describes interests that are not linked with each other. They have abrupt starts and stops, but apparently last a very long time.

Weak central coherence

Why is it called weak central coherence? It is a reference to the normally strong drive for meaning. With strong central coherence there is a pre-set preference towards perceiving wholes rather than parts. We perceive a drawing of an object and not a jumble of lines; we hear a sentence and not a jumble of words. The whole is often referred to as a Gestalt, a German term for overall form. It is used by psychologists to explain why we are normally geared to perceiving global wholes rather than local parts. However, it is only possible to show this preference when there is too much information and you can't do both at the same time.

Context is another way of describing the whole or Gestalt and its relationship to the parts. The context gives meaning to the parts. A single note of music may sound very loud when preceded by a very softly played part. The same note may sound very soft, when preceded by a loudly played part. The same is true for the pitch of tones. Absolute pitch is the ability to hear a tone exactly as it is, regardless of its context. Amazingly, about 30 per cent of individuals with autism, not trained in music, have this ability.

Weak central coherence (WCC) is a way of saying that context does not exert much force. The bits and pieces set inside a particular context are seen as what they are—the same—even if they look quite different in another context. With strong central coherence, the meaning of an element can be altered so much that it sometimes cannot be recognized as the same piece in another context. The illusion, shown in Figure 17, is a good example. Here the circle in the middle looks either big or small according to the context of the surrounding circles. Actually it is exactly the same size. If you see it as the same size, you would have demonstrated weak central coherence. You are less taken in by the illusion! Obviously, not being influenced by overall context can be a great strength. Sometimes, the word *weak* in WCC is misunderstood as meaning 'poor'. In fact most of the tests of WCC are geared to show good or superior performance.

Figure 17 also shows other visual tests, on which autistic individuals perform well. What they have in common is that they favour a strategy that automatically focuses on detail. This is the way Francesca Happé refers to it. She has done a great deal of theoretical and experimental work on this idea. For instance, she showed that this information-processing style is also typical of a proportion of the normal population, and around half of fathers and a third of mothers of autistic children.

Another task from Francesca Happé's lab is as follows. Complete the sentence: You can go hunting with a knife and ...

If you say 'fork', you have given an example of weak central coherence, in this case an association of local elements. Knife and fork go together. At the same time you have ignored the overall meaning of the sentence. If you said something like 'catch a bear', you showed evidence of strong central coherence. Another example is: 'the sea tastes of salt and ...'

Did you say 'pepper'? Again this is an example of weak central coherence. If you said something like 'fish', then you have taken the whole sentence meaning into account and this is a sign of strong central coherence.

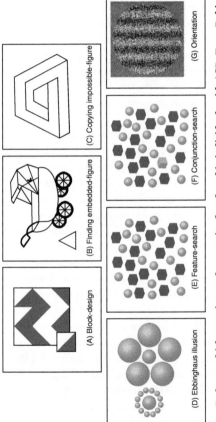

I7. Tasks on which superior perfomance is often found in individuals with ASD. From Dakin, S. & Frith, U. (2005) Vagaries of visual perception in autism. *Neuron*, 48, 497–507

According to WCC, the fourth big idea, autistic people perceive the world differently. A detail-focused processing style not only applies to vision. It also applies to hearing and to language. What about other senses—touch, for example? Here an intriguing phenomenon is that many people with autism are reported to be hypersensitive to touch. Possibly, having hyper-acute touch might be a bit like having absolute pitch.

Can weak central coherence explain savant skills? Up to a point. The ability to remember materials verbatim without understanding the content is a chief example of this style of processing information. Clearly other factors must play a role as well—practice, for instance. Repeated practice, even obsessive practice, would not be a chore for an individual who has a restricted repertoire of interests and activities. The avoidance of novelty that can be seen as typical of autism also facilitates practice. When David started to be fascinated with print, he read the *Cat in the Hat* hundreds of times. He knew it by heart, but he still reread every page of it. His ability to read words far outstripped his ability to understand them.

Weak central coherence theory tries something very daring. It tries to make sense out of a number of quite disparate aspects of autistic intelligence. It tries to account both for special talents but also for certain cognitive weaknesses. Maybe because it tries to do this all at once, it does not succeed as well as the first three big ideas we looked at, which only addressed weaknesses.

It is possible that systematic studies of attention will clarify the phenomena addressed by the weak central coherence idea. Attention to details and wholes may be quite different in nature. What happens to attention when it switches from focusing on a small element to focusing on the large whole? And vice versa? Studies suggest that autistic individuals are generally more ready to zoom in on the small element, but less able to zoom out to attend to the large whole.

Problems with the idea

Researchers have tried a number of tasks that apparently show that autistic people have no difficulty with perceiving a Gestalt. Instead there is an enhancement of the facility with which details are processed. In contrast to weak central coherence, this theory is called enhanced perceptual facilitation theory. It proposes that there is a *superiority* of detail processing in its own right, not simply a result of an *inferiority* of Gestalt processing. Systemizing is another idea that emphasizes that autistic people do not just see little details but love systems. It is this love of systems that may explain savant skills such as calendar calculation.

Another criticism is that a detail-focused processing style seems to apply only to some but not all individuals with autistic disorder. As we have seen with the other big ideas, this criticism is not necessarily fatal: none of them are likely to apply to all cases of autism spectrum disorder. There are bound to be subgroups.

Trouble at the top

It is time to turn to the last of the five big ideas, the idea of a fault in the executive system of the brain. If control is absent, then you get behaviour that is out of bounds. *You get stuck* and it is hard to get out of this. Further, you are *captured by incidentals*. You act on impulse, rather than showing foresight and planning. You don't stop and think, to find a novel solution when normal routines fail. On the other hand you *lack inhibition*, and show behaviour that is not socially acceptable. Clearly, if the executive system fails then you have problems in controlling other brain systems. This idea tries to explain the many problems that people with autism have in managing the stresses of our complex everyday life. One might have thought that such problems will only be found in low-functioning cases. But no, they are pernicious in the way they blight the lives of both low- and high-functioning people.

Gary, who was desperate to have a girlfriend, was unable to stop himself from obsessively following an attractive woman. He was told it was wrong. The woman complained to the police. He was severely reprimanded and yet his family could not trust him not to do it again. They have to closely monitor his activities. Why can he not inhibit his perfectly normal impulse?

Neuropsychologists are familiar with this sort of problem from patients with damage to the frontal lobes of the brain. Patients with frontal lobe damage are very puzzling. On ordinary IQ tests they score perfectly well, but in everyday life they make poor decisions, don't make proper plans, and generally show that they are not able to use their intelligence to adapt to their circumstances.

The role of the frontal lobes of the brain is to make high-level executive decisions. These decisions are necessary whenever routine actions are not appropriate or have to be interrupted and overridden. Here are some of the typical problems in everyday life that are all to do with trouble in this high-level control system.

Getting stuck

You cannot read a better account of this problem than the one Michael Blastland has given of his son Joe. During a long phase he would only eat one particular brand of Ricotta and Spinach pasta. He refused other food, even when he was hungry. He was so desperate about this one and only food that he could sometimes not wait for it to get cooked. Blastland also tells of Joe's insistence on watching videos over and over again. The harrowing part of this story is that Joe behaved in many ways like an addict. He craved the videos. He was inconsolable when he did not get them. And yet, when he watched them, they did not make him happy. Joe's parents were at a loss as to how to deal with these cravings and the strong dislike of anything new. Fortunately, as Joe grew up, and went to a special school, these problems lessened. Joe eventually learned to eat other foods and learned to enjoy a whole variety of activities.

Captured by incidentals

'Whenever Bob was passing a house or other building and saw an open door, he would walk through it to investigate. Needless to say, this behaviour often led to unpleasant confrontations, but apparently he was surprised every time and never learnt not to do it.' This is an example of what is often called stimulus-driven behaviour. Yet, much of our everyday perfectly normal behaviour is stimulus driven. The difference from autism is that we can keep this behaviour under control. For a person with autism it is a huge effort to inhibit certain actions when they are triggered accidentally by something that has triggered them before.

Lack of inhibition

Matthew's mother told me that she had a huge battle with him every day to get rid of rubbish. Matthew would not agree to throw anything away, not even envelopes or wrapping paper, let alone newspapers and plastic bags. This sort of problem is also sometimes seen with patients where strokes have caused lesions in the middle of the front of the brain. These patients start collecting useless things after the accident that caused their lesion. This does not mean that these particular areas of the brain are the basis of collecting behaviour. Rather, they are the basis of *inhibiting* collecting behaviour, and these patients have problems in inhibition. In the brain of rats, and presumably humans as well, there are regions deep in the brain, so-called subcortical regions, which are responsible for the drive to acquire and collect. This drive is normally controlled and kept within reasonable bounds. But this requires intact frontal lobes.

Disaster zones

Ken is stressed out when he has to do his shopping. Even though he has made a list, so as not to be tempted to buy unnecessary

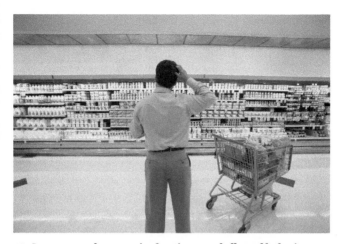

18. In a supermarket executive functions are challenged by having to plan to be within a budget; to resist impulse buying; to inhibit responses to special offers; to substitute alternatives for unavailable items. Individuals with autism find this situation very stressful, but they can follow a set routine

items, things can still go wrong. One day his brand of muesli was not on the usual shelf. Panic. Ken had no idea that it would have been perfectly alright to ask an assistant if there was some more coming in, or whether it had been put on another shelf. He had been told not to bother the assistants with questions on previous occasions. So he went home in deep frustration. This relatively mild example may give some idea how many everyday life events that demand flexibility can become major stress points. It is a peculiar lack of mental flexibility which makes their lives difficult, even in people who are otherwise very able.

Because the frontal lobes are so large and because their function is a supervisory one, the effects of damage to the frontal lobes are at once subtle and far-reaching. Impairments are found when the patients have to act spontaneously, or in a novel or unstructured situation. This is also the case for Ken. He cannot cope when his familiar routines are broken. He has been known to become violent in such situations.

Despite plentiful indicators of problems linked to poor frontal lobe function, and despite the close similarity in behaviour with frontal lobe lesion patients, no holes in the frontal lobes have ever been found in autism. There are no visible anatomical abnormalities. But the poor functioning of the frontal lobes could be due to a fault elsewhere, or a fault in connectivity with other brain regions. Investigations are in progress to find out just how the frontal lobes in autism are working during different tasks, when looked at in the scanner. One thing is clear already: they are not functioning as they should, even though they look healthy enough. They seem to be organized differently.

Problems with the idea

The idea of poor executive function is widely accepted. Further, the difficulties in everyday life are widely acknowledged to be present in most individuals with autism. But there is a major problem. The idea is so broad that it might apply to almost all neurodevelopmental disorders, not just autism.

A link between the five big ideas: a mismatch between top-down and bottom-up processes

This section is about ideas that are still only half-baked. So you need to decide whether you would like to roll up your sleeves and join me in the bakery or whether you'd rather skip to the next chapter.

Top-down and bottom-up. I like these terms and use them a lot. I think they capture something very important about how the mind/brain functions. Both these processes are necessary to perceive the world around us and above all to make sense of our perception. Here is a very simplified version of what might be happening:

Let's imagine the brain is divided into two systems. One system is geared to delivering the goods gathered from the outside world, and the other system is geared to controlling what to do next. Roughly speaking, the back of the brain is taken up by delivery processes, while the controlling system is in the front. The delivery system works bottom-up, the control system top-down. Both do a job but they must work together. Now, let's assume that in autism they do not. The proposal is that the bottom-up system is working very well, allowing superior delivery of information and superior performance on any tasks that do not involve the control system but the control system is not working well. This could be true for all of the five big ideas.

When I presented this idea at a conference, a man with Asperger syndrome came up and said he would write to me. His message was: 'Experience has told me that I should never try to understand anything. It works for neurotypicals, but you need top-down thinking to make it work. Analysis and calculation works better for us.' He had after all understood me: he likened top-down control to understanding and bottom-up delivery to analysis and calculation.

What is so important about the top-down system? There is now much evidence from the neuroscience of perception that the brain works by top-down modulation on information that enters the brain bottom-up. Not all information that enters the brain is of equal value. The top-down control system has to sort the good from the bad. It has to convey this to the delivery system. It sends signals that result in useful information being enhanced, and useless information being suppressed. One of the ways by which the top-down system controls the delivery system is through its prior expectations. These are strongly shaped by culture and our social relationships to other people. This brings in the first three big ideas.

The cook and the diner

Imagine a very choosy diner seated upstairs in the dining room, and an extremely busy cook who is doing a lot of work in the kitchen downstairs. Much of the food that the cook offers up is refused, and only choice morsels are deemed worthy of ingestion. The diner has certain preferences and naturally wishes to influence the cook to use only his favourite ingredients. He lets it be known that he is always happy to eat fresh white asparagus of the best quality. The cook, on the other hand, needs to work with the ingredients the market provides.

How does the diner communicate with the cook? By a waiter, of course. The waiter has a hard job. He has to convey to the cook the diner's extravagant orders. He also has to convey to the diner something of the reality of what is going on in the kitchen. The waiter tries to make the diner and the cook work together. He hopes that at least sometimes the diner's preferences will match the cook's speciality of the day.

The waiter has to juggle with two kinds of attention, one that is typical of the cook and one that is typical of the diner. The cook's attention arises entirely from the goods that he secures on the market. For instance, when he goes to market he will be irresistibly attracted by baskets of juicy strawberries. They will grab his attention no matter what. However, there are always many tempting ingredients that capture the cook's fancy. They are then automatically prepared the way they should be: chopped, diced, peeled, steamed, baked, boiled, or fried.

The diner's attention on the other hand, arises from the inside. He never goes to market, but he uses his memory and knowledge he gets from other diners to demand special and often novel food.

Here is an example. Another diner phones our diner and entices him to order duck eggs that are all the rage. The waiter has to spring into action and tell the cook. When the diner wants a duck egg omelette, the cook must stop using chicken eggs and spy out duck eggs.

Sometimes both are working really well together. When the cook delivers the desired omelette, the diner's enjoyment is great. Sometimes top-down attention can be in competition with bottom-up attention. The diner shouts for asparagus while the cook is preoccupied with quelling a kitchen fire. In this case the diner will not get what he desires. However, he may now order a more efficient fire extinguisher.

This parable is meant to illustrate the interplay between the brain's control and delivery systems. Neither is more important than the other. As the last example showed, the controlling system cannot override the emergency in the delivery system. However, it can take action to prevent a recurrence of the emergency. My proposal is that in autism the interplay between these two brain systems does not function well. Is this the fault of an indifferent diner, an overzealous cook, or a confused waiter? It could be any one, but personally, I tend to blame the diner.

Top-down modulation

What happens in the brain during top-down control of visual perception? A brain-imaging experiment gives some clues. In this experiment people were told in advance where to direct their attention on a screen. On the screen pairs of pictures flashed up for a split second. Importantly, the subjects could only just see them and only when they were told in advance where to look. Now the pictures were either faces or houses. This was a clever choice because the brain regions that are active when watching houses and faces are in different places. This is known from other experiments. In this experiment, when houses or faces were shown, these brain regions were indeed active too. What is more, they were more active when attention had been directed—by the experimenter's instruction—to the location where they appeared moments later. In other words, top-down attention enhances brain activity. Autistic people were scanned with exactly the same task. They showed much less enhanced activation. This is direct evidence for a lack of top-down modulation at the level of the brain in autism.

The person who has difficulty modulating attention is prone to being grabbed by external stimuli. At the same time they find it difficult to tear their attention away again. Perhaps this is why Joe eats the same food all the time; why Edward's interests are narrow and restricted; and why David has a superb but literal memory.

The absent diner

This is a rather risky idea—and I only include it because I am hoping to find an answer for the question: What is the top in top-down? My short answer at the moment is that the top in top-down is the Self. This Self is in fact the diner I have conjured up previously. The diner has certain preferences and expectations and constantly influences what is served up to him from the kitchen. So the Self has preferences and influences how the brain processes information. The diner selects what food he wishes to try. The Self decides what is of interest and what is not. An absent Self is one way to characterize the mismatch between bottom-up and top-down processing.

If there was an absent diner, then one would expect that the cook, unhampered by quirky demands from the top, would be able to produce the most gorgeous meals entirely from the ingredients to hand, and entirely doing what he is best at, by using his special skills of chopping, dicing, mashing, steaming, baking, frying. This would be one way to understand savant skills.

But isn't there a problem? What about Joe's insistence on eating exactly the same food? Does this not suggest a very strong Self? Or, in the metaphor, a diner with strongly set prior expectations? I don't think so. After all as described by Michael Blastland, there was no reasoning with Joe about this expectation. The response was impenetrably rigid. To me this suggests simple association learning or instrumental conditioning. Here the top of the command chain is an isolated but engrained response to a stimulus that has been rewarding in the past. This is the cook going it alone, doing the thing he is good at. But to no purpose because there is no diner at the top.

Here we need to recall another feature of the diner, his social interest and capacity to communicate with other diners. He does not merely make a wilful decision of what he wants to eat, but he is influenced by what other diners are eating, indeed by what is currently fashionable. We could imagine not so much an absent diner but a diner who doesn't communicate with other diners.

Some preliminary conclusions

In this chapter the non-social features of autism were in the spotlight. These include both strengths and weaknesses. The fourth idea, called weak central coherence, allowed us to celebrate the strengths of autistic people and give credit to their special talents. The fifth idea, often referred to as executive dysfunction, is concerned with their countless difficulties in managing everyday life.

I have contrasted strengths in one system of the brain—to do with delivery of information, with weaknesses in another system—to do with control of information. The evidence suggests that there is a weakness in the control system of the brain, but strength in the delivery system.

In the last part of this chapter, I have tried to speculate about a mismatch between top-down and bottom-up processes. But many questions remain open. Why are autistic people different in just the way they are? Why don't they share the social and physical world of other people? I have put the blame on the top-down controlling system of the brain, and have put the blame on an absent Self, or at least a Self that lacks normal interaction with other social beings.

Will there eventually be a satisfying formulation of the idea to explain the specifically autistic tendencies of getting stuck and lacking flexibility? Perhaps. Can the notion of the absent Self capture the autism-characteristic mismatch between top-down control and bottom-up delivery? Just possibly.

Chapter 7
From theory to practice

A trick with three boxes

In her exploration of autism, Diane surveyed many facts, saw many faces of autism, and learned about psychological experiments that have tried to penetrate deeply into the mind of the person with autism. What does it all add up to? Is there a grand unified theory? Unfortunately not. Autistic disorders are far too heterogeneous and too complex for a single satisfying account.

Nevertheless, Diane wanted to have a picture to give shape to what she has learned. She was still fascinated and now contemplated whether she should start doing some research on autism herself. With her background in natural sciences she is well equipped to pick up the necessary techniques of neuroscience. Putting together what she now knows seems a good idea. She could then see what is missing and what work needs to be done to obtain a more complete account of autism in the future.

Here is a little help. First, Diane has to tidy up the many different bits of knowledge that she has. This tidying is helped enormously by a simple trick: put different bits of knowledge into three different boxes. Let's call them *biology*, *mind*, *behaviour*. Each box is for a particular type of knowledge: in the *biology* box is knowledge gathered so far about the brain and genes; in the *mind* box are insights gained from experimental studies about the mind; and in the *behaviour* box are well-established facts about behaviour. In each box she can put lists with things she knows.

The remarkable thing that comes out of this tidying operation is that the *mind* box is the essential link between the other two. In the box for *behaviour* Diane has a list of the signs and symptoms of autism in their various and changing forms. Chapters 1 and 2 contain a lot of these facts. In the box for *biology*, she has a list of facts, some of which are presented in Chapters 3 and 4.

The *mind* box is filled with ideas that have been discussed in the last two chapters. Here we put ideas rather than facts and that is alright. The ideas are all testable and they are not taken out of the blue. They are my personal best bets for standing the test of time, and they are all backed by sound experimental studies. There are strong hints to the neural underpinnings of these features—but only hints. Diane is itching to do some of this work herself.

What we find in the biology box

For the causes of autism Diane has made a long list of factors: developmental instability, genetic predispositions, mutations, environmental risk factors, chance and accidents. These different possibilities are not exclusive and not necessarily separate from each other. Instead they may combine to lead to the large variety of disorders on the autism spectrum. As yet it seems difficult to sort out different causes at the genetic level. Different causes may affect a final common pathway, which causes similar brain-mind abnormalities and similar signs and symptoms.

Very little is as yet known about the brain in autism. Children with autism have larger brains; not at birth, but a rapid increase can be observed after the first year of life, followed by a levelling off at around eight years or so. This fact could be related to waxing and waning of neural connections: a massive proliferation of neural connections followed by savage pruning. A disturbance in these highly complex and dynamic processes might be the final common pathway of many different causes.

What we find in the behaviour box

Diane recalls that autism is currently identified by behaviour. Here she lists the core features of autism and also other features that are common, such as hypersensitivity and echoing of speech. Behavioural features are problematic because they change with age, with ability, with many factors causing differences that are not part of the underlying condition. There are no unique sets of behaviours, which will unequivocally identify autism. Two children whose autism is caused by the same biological factor may nevertheless appear different from each other. Each individual will show a different pattern of behaviour. It all depends on many factors, their own inner resources, their education, and the support they get from the outside. It is satisfying to know that a supportive educational environment can have a massive influence. It can even mask existing problems. How exactly do these influences operate? We still don't know.

What we find in the mind box

Obviously the five big ideas go into the mind box. These ideas can pull together bits and pieces lodged in the behavioural box that at first seemed unrelated. Diane knows straightaway that there would be more such ideas if she searched further. But five is a good start. The mind box would be useful as a temporary dumping ground for all the ideas and theories she would hear about autism in the future, and would invent herself. Importantly, there has to be some vetting and a need for strict testing once they are admitted. The plausible idea of a lack of social drive, the strange idea of mentalizing, and the novel idea of the broken mirror all make sense of different aspects of the hallmark of autism: the lack of reciprocal social interaction. The theory of weak central coherence tries to explain savant skills and the different way of seeing the world in general. The theory of poor executive function tries to explain all the daily difficulties in autism. All in all, the five big ideas together make sense of many of the puzzling phenomena that are thrown up by autism. Furthermore, they provide clues about the underlying neural mechanisms that might have gone wrong.

How the boxes might fit together

It is frustrating that there is no answer yet to what causes autism. There are many different risk factors, genetic and environmental. The effect of these causes is on the mind as much as it is on the brain. There might be a common pathway in the brain/mind that is ultimately affected. This would mean something quite important. Even if autism is extremely variable as far as its causes and as far as the resulting behaviour patterns are concerned, there is some common denominator. This is a cognitive phenotype. Perhaps there are more than one common pathway and more than one cognitive phenotype. This would be the case if distinct subgroups on the autism spectrum could be identified.

What if each of the five big ideas defined a cognitive phenotype? Basically you can think of a cognitive phenotype as encapsulating one of the big ideas. Perhaps this division would make the search for the causes of autism simpler. Could there be five types of autism? Possibly. But there is another possibility. The faults suggested by the five big ideas could be all mixed together like ingredients in a cake. The ingredients might be added in different quantities, and some might be optional. It is possible to imagine that different mixes would represent different points on the autism spectrum.

Let's take the example of mentalizing again. Could a mentalizing fault define a subgroup of the autism spectrum? What types of *autistic* behaviour would this explain? It could explain the core feature of an inability to engage in truly reciprocal social interaction and communication. This encompasses a big range of behaviours, which we have touched on in earlier chapters. It would fit each of our three example cases, even though David, Gary, and Edward are at very different points of the autism spectrum.

How would you identify a mentalizing fault in each case when their abilities are so varied, when the education and support they received is so vastly different? You would need a large battery of tests. And this does not exist yet. These tests have to give a choice of the right level of difficulty; they have to be reliable and they have to be ultimately linked with real-life behaviour. In principle, individual cases could be assessed using brain imaging. Given that the brain's mentalizing system has been isolated, abnormal function should be visible in this system. Existing results suggest that there should be weaker connections between the components of the system.

Let's take another example. Do David, Gary, and Edward show a cognitive phenotype of weak central coherence? This phenotype represents individuals who by preference will focus attention on details and cannot easily be distracted away. A battery of tests is again needed—tests of the right difficulty level, reliability, and validity. These would probably include tests of attention and tests of intelligence. One of the aims of the weak central coherence idea is after all to explain an uneven pattern of intelligence. We might suspect that Gary would not have this phenotype—he did not have outstanding abilities or narrow interests—but David probably would. He excelled at jigsaw puzzles, for instance. In Edward's case we might also find a big difference between his best and worst performance. Tests of signature brain activation patterns are still in the future. One might expect that they would show misconnections. This might mean too few connections between distant brain regions and too many between nearby regions. A traffic analogy comes to mind: no big highways, but a multitude of small local roads.

For Diane the boxes are beginning to fit together. Misconnections might be the reason that there is a lack of mentalizing, a lack of social drive, a broken mirror system, weak central coherence, and trouble with top-down control.

Connections and misconnections in the brain

Let's assume that in the autistic brain the wires are crossed, literally. For instance, normally, when people read minds, parts of the brain immediately get active and work in synchrony. In autism it looks as if this is not the case. Perhaps the connections between the mind-reading parts of the brain are weak precisely because there are too few of the big highway connections between these relatively distant regions, some of which are in the middle of the brain, some on the sides, and some in the back.

Autism is a neurodevelopmental disorder, which appears to be due to a disorganization of brain development. This now makes sense to Diane. But she needs another step in the argument. The disorganization might be due to lack of pruning of particular neural connections. She has to address one other issue: Why is autism apparent only from the second year of life? She asks what kinds of brain connections proliferate in the second year of life. I can only give a guess, but it could plausibly be the connections in the controlling system. From work on the visual part of the brain in animals we know that the bottom-up connections of the delivery system of the brain are ready and waiting well before the top-down connections of the controlling system are mature.

Let's assume it is the top-down connections that first proliferate and then have to be pruned. It could be that in autism precisely these connections are not cut back as quickly as they should be. If so, this would explain three things in one fell swoop: the excellent perceptual abilities of a great delivery system; the limited modulation abilities of a stalled control system, and the start of autistic symptoms in the second year. Just possibly it would also explain the bulge in brain size in autism after the first year of life.

Diane decides that a good research project would be to try and engineer a misconnected brain, for example in a mouse. How would it function? How would she test the mouse? It should have an uneven pattern of abilities. It should be able to do some tasks well, others not so well, especially tasks that need top-down control, and those that need a refined social sense.

I am delighted that Diane has decided to tackle this problem. With the right sorts of task it should be possible to show that there are systems in the brain that normally work together, but are more weakly connected in the autistic brain. I believe that in the end something has to be identified as the top in top-down, and this is what has to take the responsibility for the control. I myself have wondered whether this is a form of the Self. Is this Self absent in autism? Does this reveal a deeper meaning of the word for autism, which is after all derived from the Greek word for Self, *autos*? I cannot give an answer. However, I am looking forward with hope and fascination to the next wave of experimental investigations.

Tensions in the concept of the autism spectrum

In the course of writing this book I have been acutely aware of a tension in using examples sometimes of severe and classic cases of autism and sometimes very high-functioning cases and Asperger syndrome. There is also a gulf between the examples taken from cases of children and of adults. The anecdotes about what it feels like to be autistic all come from high-functioning adults. There is a danger therefore that the view of autism spectrum disorders is heavily weighted towards this part of the spectrum. It is not necessarily correct to call it the mild part, because these people have disabilities. They are sometimes rather thinly covered up by compensatory efforts. On the other hand, their autistic features are mild compared to the classic cases.

In the research I have reported, experiments often rely on participants with normal or high intelligence because the techniques and tasks are very demanding. These have revealed fascinating results and I make no apology for drawing on them extensively. When I remember classic cases that I know, then it seems to me that all the five big ideas are relevant to explain their behaviour, and they seem to apply simultaneously. This is not the case when I survey the high-functioning cases. Here I have the feeling that in individual cases some but not necessarily all of the big ideas are needed to explain their difficulties.

All this makes me think that it would be a good idea in future research to ask separate questions about severe autism, usually accompanied by intellectual impairment and milder forms of autism usually without intellectual impairment. It may not be possible to generalize research findings from one group to the other. The following section addresses some of the more practical questions about autism, and here it is obvious that it is necessary to treat these subgroups separately. Let's start with the highly intelligent.

Throughout this book we have had numerous occasions to look at examples of exceptional people, who have an autistic condition and who can tell us about their experiences. Temple Grandin is such a person. She has achieved accolades as a writer, presenter, and a researcher of animal behaviour. Temple Grandin's website illustrates her many astonishing talents. She can articulate what it means to have high-functioning autism and she highlights certain advantages of the thinking style, which in her own case, she describes as visual thinking. She is content to be on her own and demonstrates that it is possible to live a fulfilled life without the ability to engage in reciprocal communication. Nor is Temple Grandin the only person with autism who has written about her life, her interests, and inner experience. There are many books now by highly talented writers who reveal from a first-person point of view what it is like to have autism.

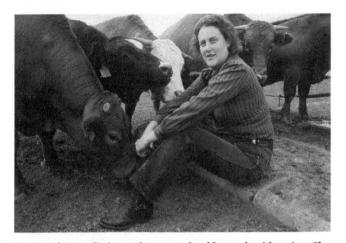

19. Temple Grandin is a spokesperson for able people with autism. She has written books on what it is like to be autistic. She designs livestock equipment and has a special affinity for animals. She wrote about this in her book, *Animals in Translation: Using the Mysteries of Autism to Decode Animal Behavior* (New York: Scribner, 2005)

If you met someone like Temple Grandin

This would be a little bit like meeting a pop star. It is more likely that you would run into someone like Edward, whose case we have looked at repeatedly. You may *not* immediately notice that Edward is 'different'. Nevertheless, for Edward to look and act normal is a tremendous effort. It may surprise you that he is very anxious, even panic stricken while you merely chat inconsequentially. In Edward's mind, anything might happen. You might suddenly turn hostile; you may suddenly make an unreasonable demand. One can make allowances for this by listening patiently and making reassuring remarks. As a rule it pays to be direct and firm. Edward would probably not take polite hints from you as signals to stop talking about bird's eggs. With luck, Edward will find a job in academia. He may even make a great discovery in a field of mathematics.

Beware. Some high-functioning persons diagnosed with an autistic condition may yet turn out not to belong to the autism spectrum but to have some other personality problem. Of course they may convince you that they have Asperger syndrome. But you can see the danger of circularity. A hard look at the boundaries of the autism spectrum will be necessary to get out of this circle.

If you met someone with autism and intellectual disabilities

Very different things would strike you when meeting Sylvia at age 40. You would know straight away that she has 'special needs'. Sylvia was a classically autistic girl who showed aloofness and insistence on sameness. She had talents as well as difficulties. She did well at a specialist school, but unfortunately, during adolescence her behaviour problems increased. She also developed epilepsy. As she became physically strong, her frustration at not understanding things often resulted in breaking things and hurting others and herself. She now needs constant supervision. Her family have no time for the notion that autism is just a difference and not a disorder. They feel this claim as cruel mockery. There is no doubt that autism has blighted Sylvia's life. But should we grieve for her and bemoan her fate? Not necessarily. Sylvia is only dimly aware of her own problems, and is as happy as anyone else who can live in a loving environment.

What about Gary? You would certainly know that there is something odd about him. You might be put off by his unkempt looks and uncouth behaviour. When you meet him, you would probably think he is a tramp. He often grumbles about not being given a fair chance, but actually, he is quite content as long as he is left in peace. Since joining the Asperger support group he has found people he feels comfortable with and counts as friends. He has even found a girlfriend among them. He may never find employment, and when he is no longer able to live at home, he will depend on social services for housing and support.

What does it cost to have an autism spectrum disorder?

Health economists make it their business to find out just how much it costs to take care of a person with an autism spectrum condition over a lifetime. In the case of Great Britain such estimates are £2.9 million for a high-functioning person with autism and £4.7 million for a low-functioning person—over a lifetime. Most of the funding currently goes on living support. However, there is less than ideal provision in many cases. The social services and special education services are chronically short of funds and could easily use more to enhance and improve their work.

It is one thing to estimate the financial burden, but the human costs are another, and cannot be estimated at all. Clearly, it is imperative to ameliorate the burden of autism.

Education and remediation

There are plenty of practical guides to educating the high-functioning and the low-functioning child respectively. Fortunately, there are effective educational programmes for children with severe autism. I have already mentioned Applied Behavioural Analysis (ABA). Here appropriate skills and behaviours are taught through learning theory principles. There is music therapy and art therapy, which are beneficial in their own right. Speech therapy can help enormously to promote articulation and the use of language. Therapies are never as easy as they sound and trained therapists are needed. A combination of several techniques is often the right answer. A gifted and committed teacher or parent makes all the difference, which is another way of saying that we don't really know what the magic ingredient is.

Some of the techniques used involve quite intense social affective interactions and games. For example, the kind of larger than life interactions enhanced by modulated voices and facial expressions that mothers use with babies. For older children and adolescents, social skills training is popular and effective. Attractive materials are available, for instance cartoons and films presenting emotional expressions in a very clear form.

One example is *Thomas the Tank Engine*, a much loved children's book, which seems to be a particular favourite with autistic children. Parents believe that the clear facial expressions on the little railway engines and the simple stories of social interactions,

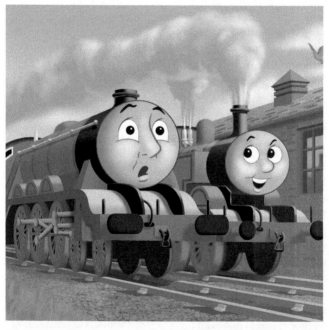

20. W. V. Awdry wrote the Railway series of books for children. *Thomas the Tank Engine* appeared first in 1946 and continues to enjoy great popularity. Autistic children are attracted to the pictures of railway engines with their big personalities and their expressive faces, and can learn about social signals through the stories

illustrating, for instance, cooperation, competition, pride, anxiety, and jealousy, are appealing enough to work as teaching aids. 'The names of the engines were the first words he used before Mum and Dad', was reported by more than one set of parents.

The Cambridge Autism Research Centre, whose website is easy to access, uses the idea of little engines, called Transporters. These heroes of tailor-made stories act as teaching aids for social skills and social signals. They show clear, simplified expressions of emotions. It is the simplicity of design and storyline that appears to enhance learning and make it enjoyable.

What kind of educational and social provisions are needed?

Deciding about education, employment, and living accommodation in later life are not one-off decisions. In discussions about the needs and rights of individuals with autism, people often get very confused because the autism spectrum is so wide. It is not possible to make general provisions that catch all. The diversity of services that are needed is enormous.

This is true for education as well. Discussions about special needs schools and integrated schooling are never ending. Parents may have strong preferences for their child to be placed in a mainstream school, thinking that this is the place where—driven by the sheer need to get along with other children—their child would be able to adapt and learn social skills. If only this were so! Instead, most children with autism seem to benefit from being taught by a specialist teacher in the calm and highly structured environment of a special unit or special school. But this is not an opinion shared by all, and the debate will continue. There are so many shades of autism that it seems sensible to make individual plans for individual children.

Medical treatments

Medical treatments for autism do not exist. However, secondary symptoms, for example, epilepsy, high anxiety, or depression, are amenable to being improved by medication. In autistic conditions, just as in typical development, it is necessary to be vigilant about all sorts of medical conditions. Many of these seem to occur unusually often in children with autism, for instance, gastric inflammation, or allergic reactions. Many of these are treatable.

If a child has gastric inflammation but does not know how to communicate this, then this child might well show a range of behaviour problems, such as biting and screaming. If the inflammation was treated with the appropriate medication, then the child would be much calmer and happier, even though the underlying problem in communication has not gone away.

Dietary interventions have their passionate proponents. Bad reactions to food allergies may well have an impact on behaviour, and taking account of these allergies makes sense. However, only some autistic children are likely to suffer from such allergies.

Charlatans

As long as there is a demand for a cure for autism, there will be people who say they can supply a cure. We certainly have no indication that autism is a disease like tuberculosis that can be cured thanks to modern pharmaceuticals. As we discussed in Chapter 4, autism is a largely genetically-based condition, with a rainbow of different facets of manifestations in behaviour. The condition is not always a disorder and not always a burden. Clearly it is absurd to wish for a cure in these cases. It is not absurd to wish for amelioration or prevention in those cases where disabilities dominate the picture. As yet, we have no proper knowledge of how to do this. Anyone who promises a short-cut, be it through taking a particular dietary supplement or other regime, should be suspected of being a charlatan. Luckily, there are websites that warn of potentially dangerous and unproven therapies.

One thing is worth knowing if you are a parent, carer, or teacher. Development is a strong force. Improvements over time, in behaviour, in social skills, and in language, are only to be expected. This is true also for the child with autism. Nothing special has to happen for these improvements to occur, over and above a typical level of care and support. This means that special interventions have to be measured against expected improvements. It is likely that educational programmes deliver significant improvements over and above these expected improvements. However, evaluating these programmes is extremely difficult. There is as yet only good practice rather than a consensus on optimal practice.

Stress

It is quite obvious that caring for a child who is unable to communicate and engage in reciprocal communication, who has rigid behaviour patterns and obsessive tendencies, is a heavy burden to bear for any family. Even in families who have vast material resources and a community network that provides services for such a child, it remains a hard task. Spare a thought also for the siblings of the child with autism.

Parents will thank you for not criticizing their methods of keeping control of tense situations. Be sympathetic when you see a family struggling to make a journey by plane, and their autistic child obsessively asks to have a drink. Yes, they probably have thought of giving him a drink! And no, they are not callous or inept. No doubt they have found out by experience that they must ignore the repeated request.

The main stress on the family is not 'what other people think'. One can get immune to raised eyebrows and know-better suggestions.

The main stress is all to do with the many open questions about autism. How frustrating it is not to know what causes the condition. If we knew, I believe parents' attitudes would change from bewilderment to a better ability to cope and to an increased chance of acceptance. Many can achieve acceptance and many gain a positive outlook, even happiness. But this is not the norm.

The effect of stress on the individual with autism is probably much worse than on healthy people. If it can be avoided, then things can go nicely in well-worked-out routines. Conversely, if there is a sudden deterioration of behaviour, look for the stress that might have caused it. So the best possible practical advice for those who are in daily contact with an autistic person is often just this: try and find out what the stressors are and remove them. They may not be obvious. For example, it may simply be an unstructured situation, as when having to make a decision of what to eat.

You don't need to be afraid of people with autism. They are different, but just like Christopher, the hero of Mark Haddon's novel, they often try very hard to be like everybody else. They might overdo it, and they may get on other people's nerves, for example, by asking strange questions at an awkward time. It is possible to cope with this better if you have gained some basic knowledge and understanding from basic research. Rather than looking for specific advice of what to say or do, which never fits the individual or the exact situation, you can formulate and think through a question yourself.

The message in this book is that scientific research has already answered some of the puzzling questions about autism and in the future will provide answers to the many questions that are still open. To decide about the proper education and care of people with autism there is no short-cut. It is essential that research is done at a very basic level, especially at the level of brain and mind.

Things we need to know more about

The puzzle of autism still beckons to be solved. In this book I have indicated black spots of ignorance in many places. Above all we need to know more about how the mind/brain works. For instance, what happens in the brain when we experience empathy, when we make eye contact, when we recognize faces, in short, when we engage in social communication with another person? We need to know more about mechanisms in the mind/brain that enable us to become aware of ourselves and of our relationship with others. Perhaps, most tantalizing of all, we need to find the secret of savant talents.

However, we can also look at these black spots of ignorance as white spots on an as-yet-unexplored continent. Explorers of all kinds, especially those who can combine psychological experiments and techniques of neuroscience, and can work hand in hand with cell biologists and geneticists, will fill in the map and will come back with answers that promise rich rewards. These answers will not only make us able to understand people with autism better, they will make us understand why all of us are who we are.

My advice to Diane is that she should not be afraid to create other big ideas and take a hard and critical look at those that are presented in this book. There is no better way to push back the frontiers of knowledge than by trying out ideas that seem a little outrageous at first—so long as they can be tested experimentally.

Specialist references

See also references cited in the captions to Figures.

On prevalence

Baird, G., Simonoff, E., Pickles, A., Chandler, S., Loucas, T., Meldrum, D., Charman, T. (2006) Prevalence of disorders of the autism spectrum in a population cohort of children in South Thames: the Special Needs and Autism Project (SNAP). *Lancet*, **368(9531)**: 210–15.

Baron-Cohen, S., Wheelwright, S., Skinner, R., Martin, J., and Clubley, E. (2001) The autism spectrum quotient (AQ): evidence from Asperger syndrome/high-functioning autism, males and females, scientists and mathematicians. *Journal of Autism and Developmental Disorders*, **31**: 5–17.

Wing, L., and Potter, D. (2002) The epidemiology of autistic spectrum disorders: is the prevalence rising? *Mental Retardation and Developmental Disabilities Research Reviews*, **8(3)**: 151–61.

On causes

Bauman, M. L., and Kemper, T. L., eds. (1994) *The Neurobiology of Autism*. Baltimore: Johns Hopkins University Press.

Courchesne, E. (2004) Brain development in autism: early overgrowth followed by premature arrest of growth. *Mental Retardation and Developmental Disability Research Reviews* **10(2)**: 106–11.

Ellman, D., and Bedford, H. (2007) MMR: where are we now? *Archives of Disease in Childhood*, **92**: 1055–7.

Geschwind, D., and Levitt, P. (2007) Autism spectrum disorders: developmental disconnection syndromes. *Current Opinion in Neurobiology*, **17(1)**: 103–11.

Gillberg, C. and Coleman, M. (2000) *The Biology of the autistic syndromes* 3rd ed. London: Mac Keith Press.

Losh, M. and Piven, J. (2007) Social cognition and the broad autism phenotype: identifying genetically meaningful phenotypes. *Journal of Child Psychology and Psychiatry*, **48(1)**: 105–12.

Minshew, N.J. and Williams D.L. (2007) The new neurobiology of autism: cortex, connectivity, and neuronal organization. *Archives of Neurology*, **64(7)**: 945–50.

Persico, A. M., and Bourgeron, T. (2006) Searching for ways out of the autism maze: genetic, epigenetic and environmental clues. *Trends in Neuroscience*, **29(7)**: 349–58.

Rutter, M. (2006) *Genes and Behavior: Nature-Nurture Interplay Explained*. Oxford: Blackwell.

Yeo, R. A., Gangestad, S. W., and Thoma, R. J. (2007) Developmental instability and individual variation in brain development: implications for the origin of neurodevelopmental disorders. *Current Directions in Psychological Science*, **16**: 245–9.

On impairments of social interaction

Baron-Cohen, S., Tager-Flusberg, H., and Cohen, D., eds. (2000) *Understanding Other Minds: Perspectives from Developmental Cognitive Neuroscience*. Oxford: Oxford University Press.

Dapretto, M., Davies, M. S., Pfeifer, J. J., Scott, A. A., Sigman, M., Bookheimer, S. Y. *et al.* (2006) Understanding emotions in others: mirror neuron dysfunction in children with autism spectrum disorders. *Nature Neuroscience*, **9(1)**: 28–30.

Dawson, G., Meltzoff, A. N., Osterling, J., Rinaldi, J., and Brown, E. (1998) Children with autism fail to orient to naturally occurring social stimuli. *Journal of Autism and Developmental Disorders*, **28(6)**: 479–85.

Hirschfeld, L., Bartmess, E., White, S., and Frith, U. (2007). Can autistic children predict behavior by social stereotypes? *Current Biology*, **17(12)**: R451–2.

Mundy, P., and Newell, L. (2007) Attention, joint attention and social cognition. *Current Directions in Psychological Science*, **16(5)**: 269–74.

Pelphrey, K., Morris, J. P., McCarthy, G. (2005) The neurological basis of eye gaze processing deficits in autism. *Brain*, **128** (Pt 5): 1038–48.

Rizzolatti, G., Fogassi, L., Gallese, V. (2006) Mirrors of the mind. *Scientific American*, **295(5)**: 54–61.

Rogers, S., and Williams J. H. G., eds. (2006) *Imitation and the Social Mind: Typical Development and Autism*. New York: Guilford Press.

On non-social features

Bird, G., Catmur, C., Silani, G., Frith, C., Frith, U. (2006) Attention does not modulate neural responses to social stimuli in autism spectrum disorders. *Neuroimage*, **31(4)**: 1614–24.

Gilbert S.J., Bird G., Brindley R., Frith C.D. and Burgess P.W. (2008) Atypical recruitment of medial prefrontal cortex in autism spectrum disorders: An fMRI study of two executive function tasks, *Neuropsychologia*, **46(9)**: 2281-91.

Happé, F., and Frith, U. (2006) The weak central coherence account: detail focused cognitive style in autistic spectrum disorders. *Journal of Autism and Developmental Disorders*, **36**: 5–25.

Heaton, P., Williams, K., Cummins, O., and Happé, F. (2007) Autism and pitch processing splinter skills: a group and subgroup analysis. *Autism*, 12: 203–19.

Hermelin, B. (2001) *Bright Splinters of the Mind: A Personal Story of Research with Autistic Savants*. London: Jessica Kingsley.

Hill, E.L. (2004) Executive dysfunction in autism. *Trends in Cognitive Sciences*, **8(1)**: 26–32.

Mann T.A. and Walker P. (2003) Autism and a deficit in broadening the spread of visual attention, *Journal of Child Psychology and Psychiatry*, **44(2)**: 274–84.

Mottron, L., Dawson, M., Soulieres, I., Hubert, B., and Burack, J. (2006) Enhanced perceptual functioning in autism: an update, and eight principles of autistic perception. *Journal of Autism and Developmental Disorders*, **36(1)**: 27–43.

Further reading

Classic readings

Asperger, H. (1944) Die 'autistischen Psychopathen', in *Kindesalter*, trans. U. Frith in U. Frith, ed. (1991) *Autism and Asperger Syndrome*. Cambridge: Cambridge University Press.

Kanner, L. (1943) Autistic disturbances of affective contact, *Nervous Child*, **2**: 217–50.

Introductions

Frith, U. (2003) *Autism: Explaining the Enigma*. Oxford: Blackwell.

Medical Research Council UK (2001) *Autism: Research Review*, MRC website.

Sigman, M., and Capps, L. (1997) *Children with Autism: A Developmental Perspective*. Cambridge, Mass.: Harvard University Press.

Houston, R., and Frith, U. (2002) *Autism in History*. Oxford: Blackwell.

Morton, J. (2004) *Understanding Developmental Disorders: A Cognitive Modelling Approach*. Oxford: Blackwell.

Edited volumes presenting research

Charman, T., and Stone, W., eds. (2006) *Social and Communication Development in Autism Spectrum Disorders: Early Identification, Diagnosis, and Intervention*. New York: Guilford Press.

Frith, U., and Hill, E., eds. (2003) *Autism: Brain and Mind*, Oxford: Oxford University Press.

McGregor, E., Nunez, M., Cebula, K., and Gomez, J. C. *et al.*, eds. (2008) *Autism: An Integrated View from Neurocognitive, Clinical and Intervention Research*. Oxford: Wiley-Blackwell.

Volkmar, F. R., Paul, R., Klin, A., and Cohen, D. J., eds. (2005) *Handbook of Autism and Pervasive Developmental Disorders, Diagnosis, Development, Neurobiology, and Behavior*, 3rd edition. Hoboken, NJ: Wiley.

Biographical accounts

Claiborne-Park, C. (1967, 1995) *The Siege*. New York: Little Brown.

Blastland, M. (2006) *Joe: The Only Boy in the World*. London: Profile Books.

Grandin, T. (1996) *Thinking in Pictures: My Life with Autism*. New York: Vintage Books.

Lawson, W. (2000) *Life behind Glass: A Personal Account of Autism Spectrum Disorder*. London: Jessica Kingsley.

Moore, C. (2004) *George and Sam*. London: Penguin.

Sacks, O. (1995) *An Anthropologist on Mars*. New York: Vintage Books.

Guide books

Attwood, T. (2006) *A Complete Guide to Asperger's Syndrome*. London: Jessica Kingsley.

Siegel, B. (2003) *Helping Children with Autism Learn: Treatment Approaches for Parents and Professionals*. Oxford: Oxford University Press.

Wing. L. (1997) *The Autism Spectrum: A Guide for Parents and Professionals*. London: Constable.

Index

Autism

Index

INTELLIGENCE
A Very Short Introduction
Ian J. Deary

Ian J. Deary takes readers with no knowledge about the science of human intelligence to a stage where they can make informed judgements about some of the key questions about human mental activities. He discusses different types of intelligence, and what we know about how genes and the environment combine to cause these differences; he addresses their biological basis, and whether intelligence declines or increases as we grow older. He charts the discoveries that psychologists have made about how and why we vary in important aspects of our thinking powers.

'There has been no short, up to date and accurate book on the science of intelligence for many years now. This is that missing book. Deary's informal, story-telling style will engage readers, but it does not in any way compromise the scientific seriousness of the book . . . excellent.'

Linda Gottfredson, University of Delaware

'Ian Deary is a world-class leader in research on intelligence and he has written a world-class introduction to the field . . . This is a marvellous introduction to an exciting area of research.'

Robert Plomin, University of London

www.oup.co.uk/isbn/0-19-289321-1

DRUGS
A Very Short Introduction
Leslie Iverson

The twentieth century saw a remarkable upsurge of research on drugs, with major advances in the treatment of bacterial and viral infections, heart disease, stomach ulcers, cancer, and mental illnesses. These, along with the introduction of the oral contraceptive, have altered all of our lives. There has also been an increase in the recreational use and abuse of drugs in the Western world. This book explains what drugs are, how they work, and how medicines are developed and tested. It also discusses current ideas about why some drugs are addictive, and whether drug laws need reform.

> 'extremely interesting and capable ... although called a very short introduction, it contains a wealth of information for the interested layman and is exemplary in its accuracy.'
>
> **Malcolm Lader, King's College, London**

> 'a slim but assured and wise volume on drugs. [It] takes up many controversial positions ... with an air of authority that commands respect. It is difficult to think of a better overview of the field for anyone new to it.'
>
> **David Healy, University of Wales College of Medicine**

www.oup.co.uk/isbn.0-19-285431-3

PSYCHOLOGY
A Very Short Introduction
Gillian Butler and Freda McManus

Psychology: A Very Short Introduction provides an up-to-date overview of the main areas of psychology, translating complex psychological matters, such as perception, into readable topics so as to make psychology accessible for newcomers to the subject. The authors use everyday examples as well as research findings to foster curiosity about how and why the mind works in the way it does, and why we behave in the ways we do. This book explains why knowing about psychology is important and relevant to the modern world.

'a very readable, stimulating, and well-written introduction to psychology which combines factual information with a welcome honesty about the current limits of knowledge. It brings alive the fascination and appeal of psychology, its significance and implications, and its inherent challenges.'

Anthony Clare

'This excellent text provides a succinct account of how modern psychologists approach the study of the mind and human behaviour. ... the best available introduction to the subject.'

Anthony Storr

www.oup.co.uk/vsi/psychology